SPORTS, EXERCISE and ASTHMA

A Solution to the Clinical Sand Traps of Allergic and Asthmatic Disease

All About Allergy
Looking Well and Feeling Well

THE THOUGHT BEHIND THE SHOT

Sports Exercises Illustrated By The Leading Sports Artist, LeRoy Neiman

Leonard S. Girsh, M.D

LEONARD S. GIRSH, M.D.

Sports, Exercise and Asthma

Library of Congress Catalog Card Number 2011963657

The Thought Behind The Shot™ is a trademark of Leonard S. Girsh, M.D.

Thought Behind The Shot™ is a trademark of Leonard S. Girsh, M.D.

Art of the Book Cover:

Westchester Golf Club
copyright © LeRoy Neiman, Inc. 1979

Note: The information in this book can be a valuable addition to your doctor's advice, but it is not intended to replace the services of trained health professionals. You are advised to consult with your doctor regarding matters relating to your health, particularly regarding symptoms that may require immediate attention.

ISBN-13: 978-1500928681

ISBN-10: 1500928682

PRINTED IN U.S.A

OUR GOAL

"The thought of being able to engage a child or an adult, in chronic care self management goals, using a favorite sport related warm-up exercise is brilliant in its simplicity and yet can be comprehensive in its outcome." Mark Sobiski, Development Manager Care South Carolina Inc.

DEDICATION

The Thought Behind the Shot is dedicated to the asthmatic children who faithfully helped initiate and successfully benefited from the physical conditioning program that came from a blend of principals of play and exercise coupled with the much revered motivational spirit, force and excitement that great American sports offer and the great masterpieces of sports created from the brush of the artist, **LeRoy Neiman**.

When children in other clinics appealed to me for admission, patients in multiple clinics appreciating the benefits of good health, I realized that this advance and exercise therapeutics should be broadened and entitled "Sports, Exercise, and Health" as it specifically enhances efficiency in the respiratory system and oxygenation, looking at the respiratory system as a pump aided by the efficiency provided by the sports warm-up exercises as if training for the Olympics of health, as Mark Sobiski notes, making oxygenation more efficient in aiding recovery.

Then realizing that this is augmenting as a broncho-pulmonary thoracic pump for oxygenation the patients artfully led us to this broad-spectrum usage in advancing sports in exercise regarding health, building on our original plan and successful results for asthma.

As you can see by our goal, the book is so directed, as quoted by Mark Sobiski as well as the White House augmenting Mrs. Michelle Obama's work, to increase activity and advance diet to counter obesity.

This book describes readily adaptable everyday care to improve the health in a child or adult. The use of these non-invasive techniques of breathing would benefit all of us but particularly focuses on preparing a patient to calmly cope with an impending or possible threatening, such as an asthma attack. This recognizes the importance of oxygen flow and its delivery in the reconstitution of tissue in everyday metabolism as well as meeting the challenges of healing.

The ingenuity provided here resulted from the efforts of a team of physicians, sports educators, enthusiastic children and adults imbued with the winning team spirit found in sports.

Making a wish come true:

This book is the result of patients making a wish to the physician. It allows for simplicity of achievement wherein they are able to partake in sports without the impairment of asthma that would interfere with their physical activity. This concept is also similarly intriguing for adults, because we are all dedicated to these heroes of the sports arena.

Several children appealed to us, apologetically, asking if even though they didn't have asthma, and could they be a member of this motivational sports rehabilitation program. I responded, "Just asking to be a member was more than enough, please join us."

The Art of Medicine

&

Medical Care in Art

The choreography of the rhythmic form, chest physiotherapy as remarkably viewed in sports paintings by **LeRoy Neiman**

The White House, through Michelle Obama, regarding her national campaign to increase activity and advance diet to counter obesity in children, appreciated that *Sports, Exercise and Health* be used in this national presentation. Conditioning, using this application technology, can prepare a patient to prevent an asthmatic attack. Breathing exercises and warm-up exercises of their sport of choice enhances the function and activation of the sensory muscles and respiration of the asthmatic child. Based on the observation that musicians playing wind instruments rarely had asthma, this gives the additional positive effects of these exercises.

THE WHITE HOUSE
WASHINGTON

We would like to extend our deepest thanks and appreciation for your generous gift.

It is gratifying to know that we have your support. As we work to address the great challenges of our time, we hope you will continue to stay active and involved.

Again, thank you for your kind gift.

WWW.WHITEHOUSE.GOV

FOREWORD

When I first met the author I was impressed with his professional and intellectual competence and particularly his dedication to the best of care for his patients. Dr. Girsh consequently developed an interdisciplinary approach to improving the health and well being of children whose allergies contribute to asthma and other breathing difficulties. Over the period of the approximate three years that my graduate students and I associated with the program, we became more aware and appreciative of the developed interdisciplinary approach undertaken.

Discussions with professionals with wide divergent backgrounds helped us learn about the needs of children with asthma from different perspectives. This approach to health care seemed exciting for all of those involved. As an exercise physiologist, my focus started primarily with an emphasis on exercise as a process to improve the physical and mental health of the children. As the hours of contact with the children and the hours of discussions with professionals in other disciplines increased, my focus became much wider. I believe most of the other people involved with the care of the children similarly became more broadly focused. This seemed especially true for Dr. Girsh who was responsible for the coordination of the group as well as the care of the children.

The excitement of the staff as well as the participating children seemed to increase weekly as the interactions continued with the purpose of helping the patients improve. The children seemed to be able to do more without hesitancy and their positive outlook regarding themselves was usually increased. This conclusion broadens the application of this technology to many illnesses.

This program had and has a broad appeal to many ill children, e.g. some children from other clinics wanted to be in the program as well and this added to our realization of its broad application and appeal.

The emphasis: To help children as well as adults move towards normal, functional behavior particularly when coordinated with the rest of their medical care. This sets an attainable goal of better health.

The procedures recommended in this text clearly contribute to this goal.

Arne Olson, Ph.D.,
Former Professor, Dept. of Sports and Physical Education, Temple University, Philadelphia, PA
Former Professor and Chairman, Dept. of Physical Education, East Stroudsburg, PA

LEONARD S. GIRSH, M.D.

Table of Contents

INTRODUCTION

THE THOUGHT BEHIND THE SHOT

"A Problem is an Opportunity in Work Clothes"

This book corresponds to the Olympics best illustrated by a USA gold medalist, an asthmatic youth, who took seriously the challenge of asthma, a breathless disease. In training for this achievement she utilized her buoyancy in the water to facilitate strengthening and developing her accessory muscles of respiration. It is this example that motivated the children to adopt warm-up exercises of the sport of their choice to better condition their accessory muscles of their chest bronchopulmonary pump, incorporating their Olympic challenge of training to best cope with an asthma attack using these preventative measures.

The water and its humidified clear air (as if filtered) and the short spurts of her swimming specialty, (the 100 meter breast stroke which she completed with the record time of 1 minute, 7.05 seconds, helps provide the feeling of euphoria in winning and being "on top of the world"). The first four minute peak of exercise provides the body`s own adrenaline, a bronchodilator which counteracts the bronchial spasm of asthma, produced under the stimulus of her exercise program. The team coach then applies these observations and guidance in programming the asthmatic patient's sports involvement until more prolonged exercise tolerance is achieved.

Several other Olympic Gold medalists can be added to this list, substantiating that the physical accomplishments and potential physical accomplishments in sports and other fields of endeavor are achievable in such common bronchopulmonary diseases as asthma emphasizing the need for companion sports oriented chest physiotherapy programs. Asthma formerly had an incidence of 3 to 5 percent of the population, but this incidence has doubled making it one out of every nine people having asthma at some point in their lives. In certain areas of the country the incidence is even greater.

One of our very prominent citizens, at the beginning of the 20th century, and one of our American presidents with bronchial asthma, Teddy Roosevelt, was probably one of the earliest to pioneer physical fitness, as a helpful and healthful addition in the management of one's own bronchial asthma.

Little did he know how far reaching he would be in his physical fitness program. How popular and valuable it would become in physical conditioning the asthmatic individual, (a campaign continued 50 years later by Pres. John F. Kennedy). We have enabled the child or adult with an acute asthma attack or chronic asthma to better able cope with his or her problem. Little did the former president know the emphasis leading to the discovery of the importance of the body's lymphatic cleansing system through the pump-like action of breathing exercises and the cleaning mechanisms thereby of breathing. Therefore it is an important addition in cardiac disease and cardiopulmonary disease.

Improvement in the first four minutes of exercise in the asthmatic patient has never been stressed. I have repeatedly documented, with comparative pulmonary function testing before and after 4 minutes of exercise, as a respiratory stress test, that the majority of asthmatics can improve when so stressed with major physical exertion in the first four minutes of strenuous exercise. **After the asthma is under good control, including a sports exercise program, with therapeutics presented in concert with strategic avoidance of two or three key allergens based on immunologic studies, as well as with appropriate desensitization and medication, such as bronchodilator so that longer spurts of exercise may ultimately be achieved, progressively, as tolerated. These goals are all accomplished within the range of adequate rest and good diet as part of the program.**

Exercise and diet represent the new advances in therapeutics, but must be used with the well established management of specific diseases, such as obesity in children, pioneered by President and Michelle Obama. Therapeutic specificity can be used such as for the metabolic syndrome of obesity.

Unique to this program is that the patient selects a favorite sport in which he or she would like to participate and this goal can be kept in mind while we incorporate the necessary breathing exercises, postural drainage, pursed lip breathing exercises amongst others, all so helpful in augmenting the broad three-prong approach to healthcare. In addition to these exercises, adequate rest and diet individually directed to the allergy and asthmatic disease should be included.

Identifying and minimizing the target offending and aggravating key factors to avoid or more practically, to minimize, is to be selectively considered. At the same time, designing and administering a vaccine to build the patient's immune system.

Sports, Exercise and Asthma allows us to best appreciate and incorporate into our exercise and diet in building our final treatment program. This will allow us to achieve our treatment goal in allergic and asthmatic allergic disease management to achieve our final goal of looking well and feeling well.

These principals are looked upon as helping to minimize the allergic load while building up the patient's resistance to allergy.

The approach to any disease can be looked upon in the same fashion.

Smooth Sailing

The imaging of such positive sports settings as swimming and floating on a lake or ocean along with inhaling all the clean air around the lake area, is helpful in overcoming various degrees of acute and even severe asthma.

Breathing the clear air of a nearby lake or ocean is coupled with the relaxing scene and wish for "Smooth Sailing" as depicted in the painting. This painting, a signed original hanging in my consultation room, cheerfully reinforced my care individually and specifically for each patient. Jogging at the beach at the peak of the noonday sun offers air over the water that is clear of pollen, mold, and dust and can be enjoyed by all and well appreciated by the asthmatic patient. (The sun also lessens possible chill or cold air to be minimized by the asthmatic.)

This conveys our wish to the patient of smooth sailing, with the illness of asthma being the stormy seas, presented in the associated art format based on the statement that "a picture is worth a thousand words".

The patient can picture relaxed inhalation of the clear air of the seashore.

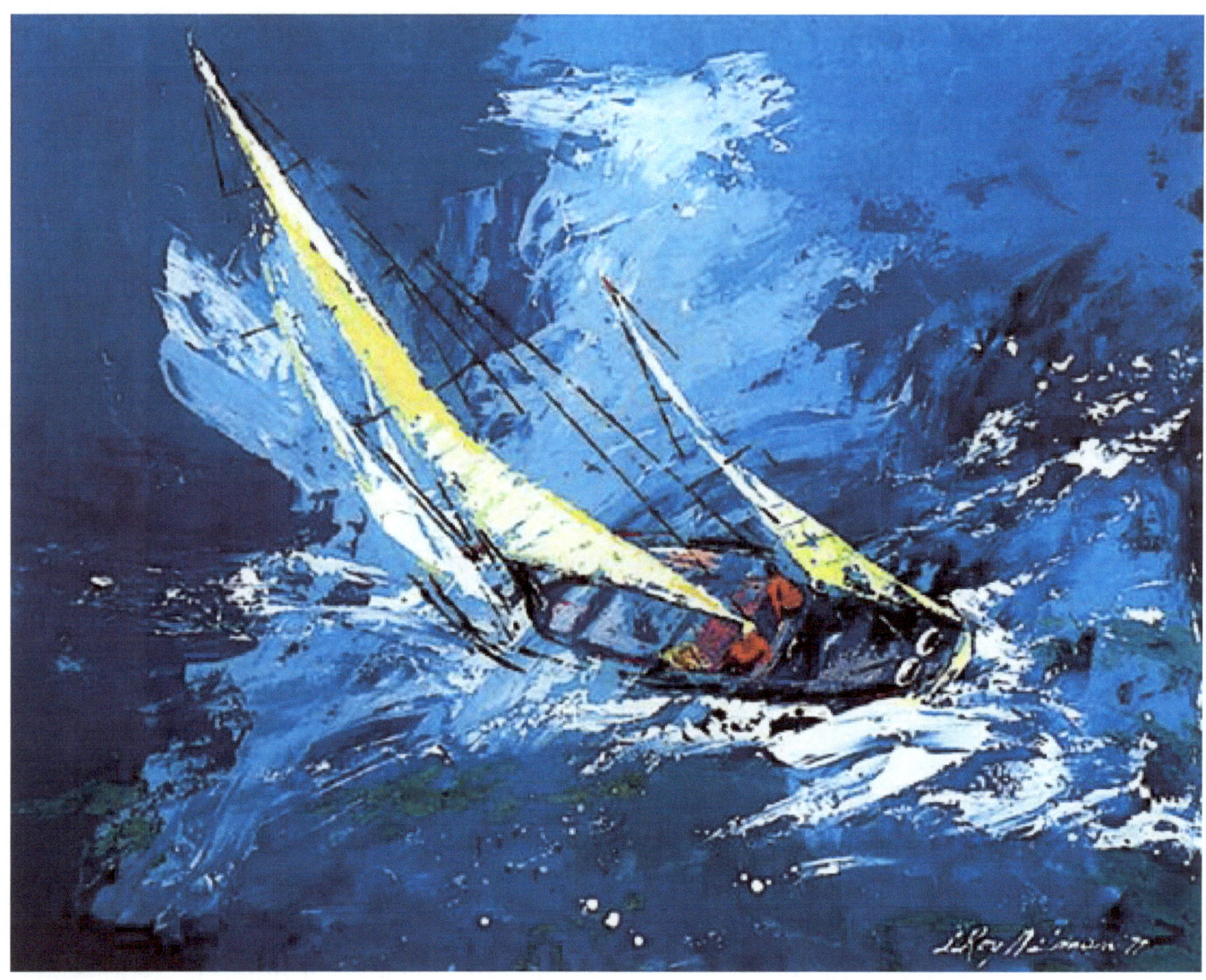

Sailing

copyright © LeRoy Neiman, Inc. 1977

"Smooth Sailing"

Celebrated Classic Sports art by LeRoy Neiman, presented here for specialized health care medical application with the artist's personal permission.

The program was developed and utilized by the author, Dr. Leonard S. Girsh, in his private practice and clinic. As director of the Allergy and Asthma Dept. and residency program of Temple University Medical Center Children's Hospital, in conjunction and close cooperation with Asthmatic Center/ Children Heart Hospital, also founded by Dr. Girsh, along with the pediatric allergy residency program, with the Physical Education Dept. also of Temple University, was initially used as a pediatric program and later extended to all ages. Sports exercises as in all aspects of health care represent a mind-body integrative program with all the cultural reinforcements of great art.

A creative selective, collection, correlation and adaptation of the best of art depicting various sports by **LeRoy Neiman** with the best of breathing exercises and chest physiotherapy for bronchopulmonary disease initiated first in children, now applicable to all ages with diseases such as asthma, emphysema, chronic bronchitis, and cystic fibrosis.

The author has incorporated all of these disciplines:

Sports, art, physical education and music are used here in the management of respiratory allergy and asthma in conjunction with chest physiotherapy is discussed here. These methods also include positive imaging such as relaxed breathing in a peaceful setting or of breathing the clean cool air around a lake or pool. A technique of relaxed pursed lip breathing for asthma flare ups, even if medications were forgotten or momentarily unavailable is illustrated in this text. A technique of selecting sports utilizing brief spurts or bursts of exercise e.g. tennis, baseball pitching and batting, and point counting for basketball scoring practice (the well known game of 21).

It is advisable to select an indoor sport environment for the pollen and mold allergic patient. Indoor warm-up exercises for basketball, techniques of tennis, swimming, dancing, and rope jumping might be appropriate choices. The practice components of the above sports can be incorporated with and be an integral part of exercise conditioning of the accessory muscles of respiration. Elbow and shoulder circling, abdominal breathing exercises, pursed lip breathing, and general body conditioning should also be part of the program.

Enthusiasm and the spirit of winning and achievement so evident in all sports help participants develop a positive attitude that we like to incorporate in working towards recovery in asthma with all the therapeutic methods available for bronchial asthma.

The selection of above sports where there are short bursts of exercise of less than 4 minutes can help open the airway until asthma is under control.

Sports exercises that involve 8 or more minutes of continued running or exercising might then be considered when the asthma is under <u>good</u> <u>control,</u> with the supervised review of your physician and with comparative pulmonary function testing before and after the 8 minutes of running or exercise, such as cross country running, or the constant running and jumping sports of basketball and soccer. I have been able to document, by repeated pulmonary function testing, that the asthma remains under good control after the 8 minutes of exercise.

The following exercises incorporate shoulder girdle exercises with exercises of the other accessory muscles of respiration including muscles of the neck and thorax:

These are the accessory muscles of respiration that help to stabilize the chest during acute asthma. For example, in acute severe asthma, the patient usually leans forward to breathe more comfortably and strains neck, shoulder and chest muscles (all the accessory muscles of respiration) and holds on to the arms of the chair to stabilize these accessory muscles of respiration. This same straining of accessory muscles of respiration can be seen in the runner, ready to break the tape at the end of the race.

They are using all of their energies to win the race. (See art work depicting soccer players), becoming increasingly popular in the United States. The asthmatic patient gives the same appearance sitting still.

In his autobiography, Armand Hammer describes an acute asthma attack very well when he writes of a meeting with Chernenko, during which time the Russian leader had a broncho-spasm attack, precipitated by the very cold air of Russia and tobacco smoke.

SPORTS, EXERCISE AND ASTHMA

Sports Rx, chest physiotherapy, helps to condition and build stamina to these respiratory muscles. The patient is guided and encouraged to select the sports exercise group as determined by his or her favorite sports interest.

1. **Swimming, boating and nautical sports**: Swimming is the best tolerated exercise for the asthmatic patient. With swimming, buoyancy and weightlessness enhance muscle relaxation. The water actually can help wash away some of the effects from exposure to pets, pollen or mold. The technique of washing away allergens with warm water – washing hands, face, nostrils while showering is most helpful. Humidity is helpful in asthma and moisture minimizes air-borne pollen, mold and dust inhalants. The Australian crawl, breaststroke, side and back strokes, involve elbow and arm circling. Use of the hair dryer is important after swimming during cold weather, especially for patients prone to recurrent upper respiratory infection. Cautionary steps should be used with chlorinated water - swim only prior to additional chlorination.

2. Scoring of **baskets in basketball**.

3. **The driving range for golf as well as the game of golf.** (as shown on the front cover). **Golf is an extremely popular and dedicated sport in Japan.**

4. **Baseball and softball catching, throwing and pitching practice, the stretching and reaching of outfield and in field fielding practice, batting practice. (Fig. 1)**

5. **The football catch and touch football. (Fig. 2)**

6. **Tennis, volleyball serve and 4 point Wimbledon tennis.**

7. **Volleyball.**

8. **Running or jumping rope.**

9. **Bowling.**

18

The ABCs of Sports and Physical Education

Throwing, catching and batting – Most sports are developed from these themes. Illness often interferes with learning and fully developing sports skills so celebrated in this country and worldwide. These skills are important for asthmatic children as well as others.

In healing as in medicine we like to address and correct all of the deficiencies in treating the whole person. In our program, by incorporating chest physiotherapy with sports exercise we are doing both.

Physical conditioning principles for asthmatic as well as others emphasize the specific components of physical fitness. The components are strength, muscular endurance, circulatory-respiratory endurance and flexibility.

Strength training focus is on progressive resistance exercise for specific muscle groups. Six to ten repetitions maximum are guidelines. Each muscle group is exercised for brief periods which should be adapted to each individual and to be within the reach of the asthmatic. General fatigue is not to be reached. Our goal is to build up progressive endurance, as tolerated, with particular emphasis on the sports of the child's or adult's choice and with particular emphasis on breathing exercises associated with that sport.

SPORTS, EXERCISE AND ASTHMA

BASEBALL- The great American sport and little league goal of every child:

If the child selects baseball as an activity, the following diagram is an example of warm-up exercises specific to this sport. If we picture an asthmatic patient, they prefer to sit anxiously forward in a chair, grasping the arms of the chair, while fixating the muscles in the shoulder girdle, chest, neck, and supporting back muscles. In all actuality, this may be looked upon as conditioning not only for the sport of choice, but also as if the patient was training for the Olympics as an asthmatic enabling them to use the exercises each day. This may be part of the whole picture of care. If done alone (even though we don't advise it) would also be helpful though not ideal. A sports physician can be reached to complete this care.

Baseball

Baseball warm up exercises are representative of very pleasant accessory respiratory muscular exercises.

Warm up exercises of baseball and softball, catching, throwing and pitching practice, the stretching and reaching of outfield and infield fielding practice, and batting practice.

The artful skills of throwing a baseball, basketball or football, can be well utilized as a companion to chest physiotherapy program performed with team mates - Little League or the camaraderie of our family, friends and neighbors.

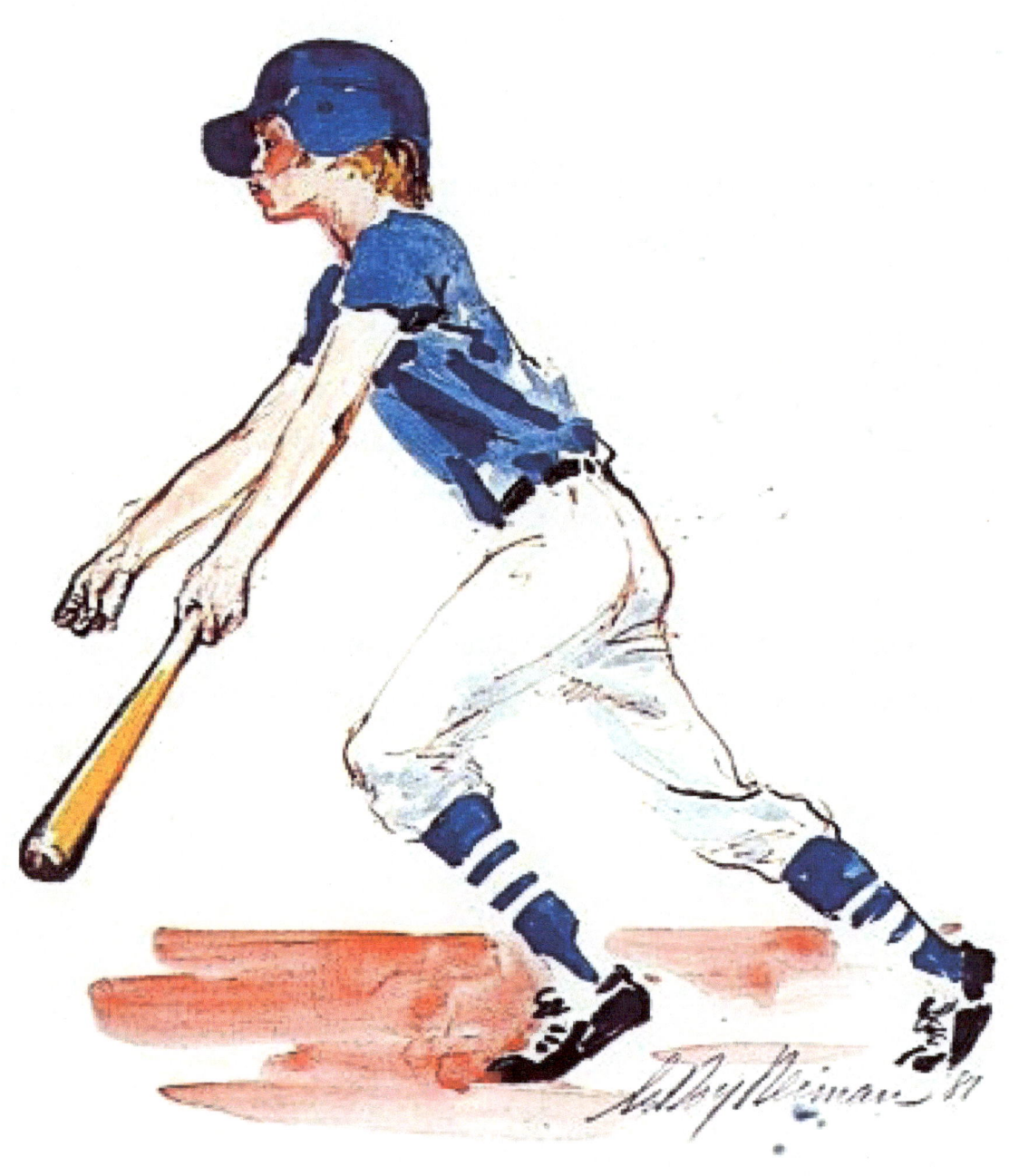

Little Hitter

22

Still, many children have not had the opportunity to participate in physical activities due to sickness. Sports and other physical activities may be a great value to children and young adults.

In my personal experiences, I have witnessed children who were not diagnosed as asthmatics were very much enthused to participate in my physical activities catered towards asthmatic patients. During the activities all the children participated and were treated equally, not discriminated upon due to their disease. The spirit of winning or achieving plays an integral part of increasing the overall quality of life.

This is the same enthusiastic spirit we would like to implement into the patients overall recovery. In sharp contrast to medicine alone, sports and physical activity builds up the patients resistant, allowing the patient to strive to lessen the need for medication. This should be looked upon as a very valuable addition to your doctor's advice, not intended to replace the services of trained health professionals. Always use in conjunction with his advice.

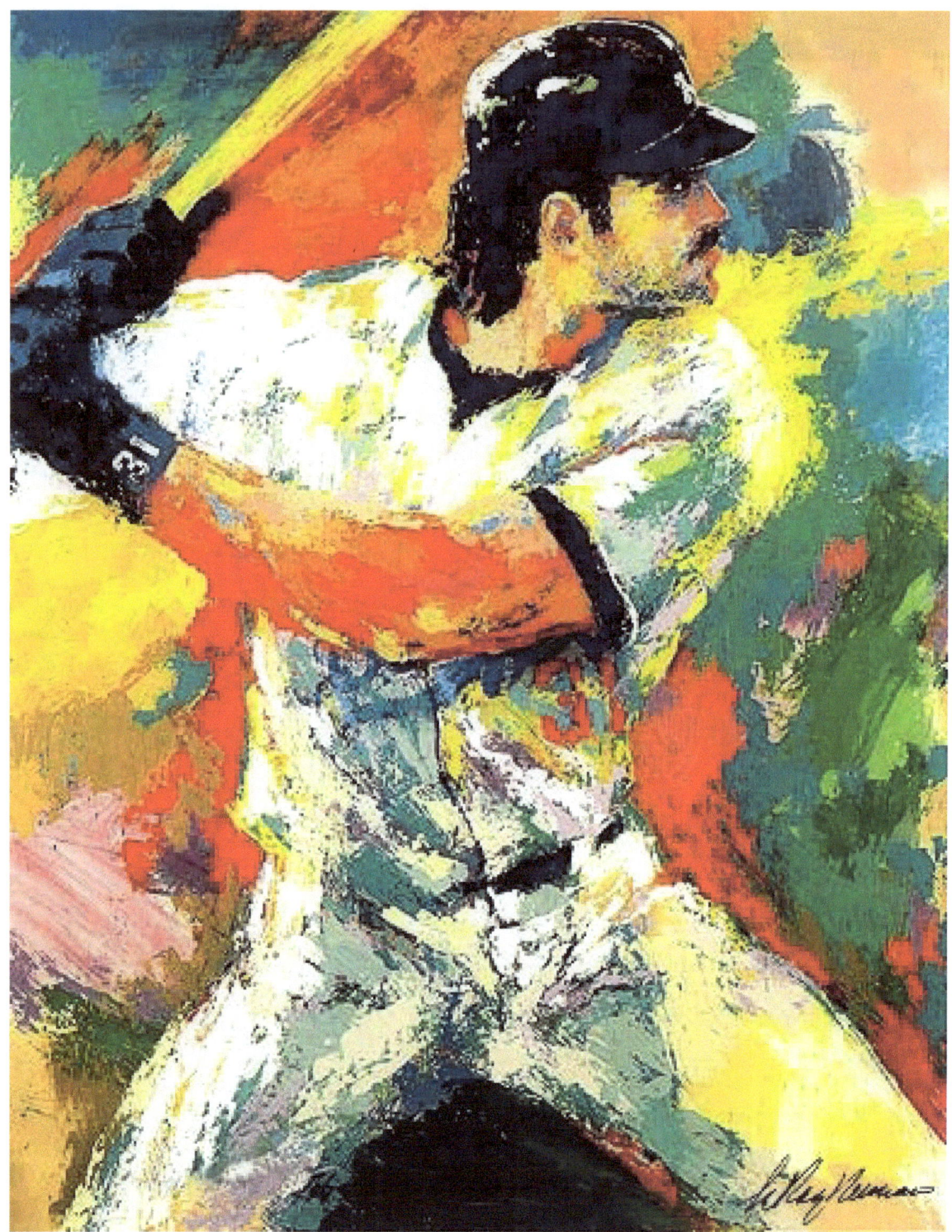

Mike Piazza

The ABC's of a sports exercise program as taught to us by the nation's leaders in baseball.

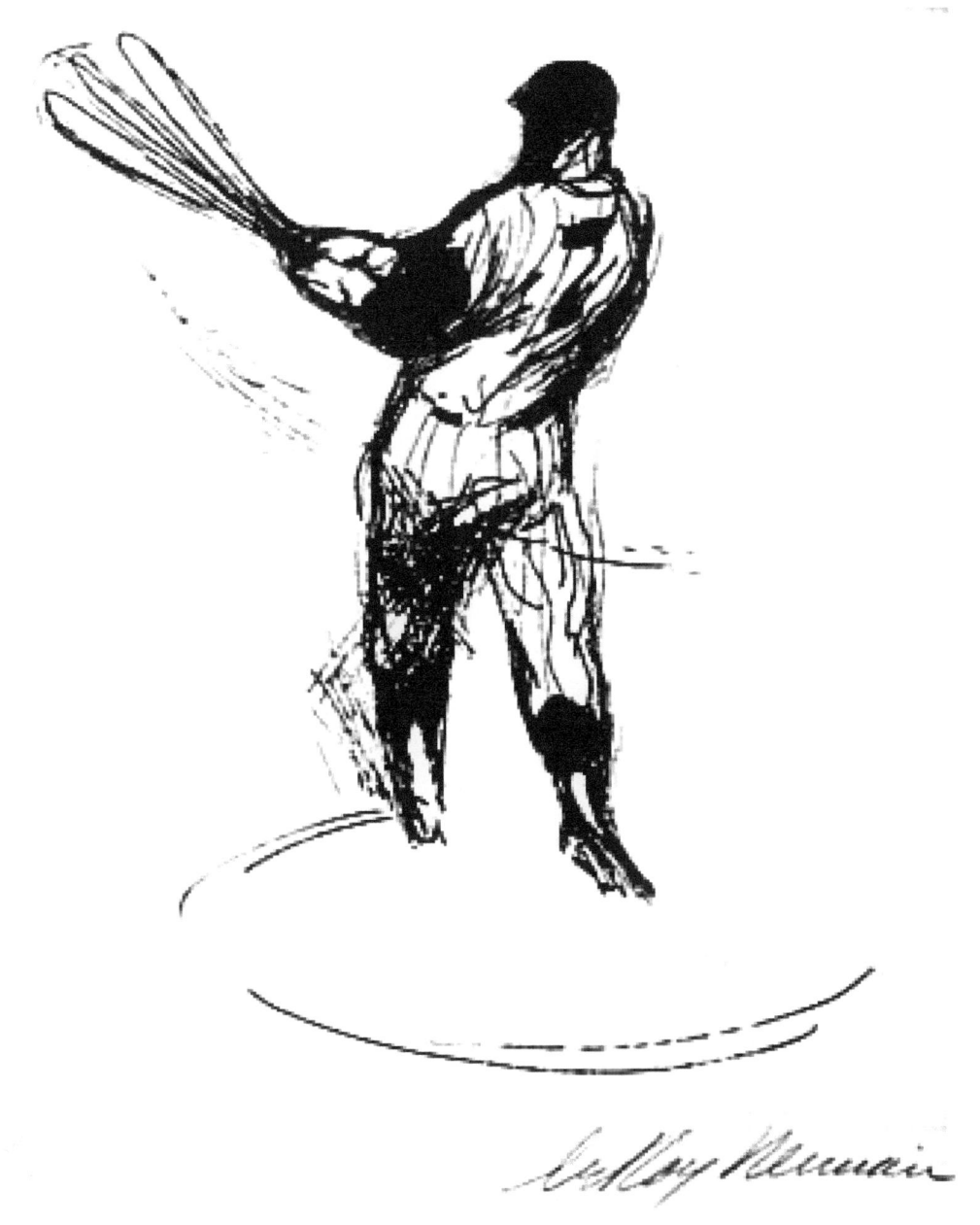

Warm-up Swing, Mickey Mantle

copyright © LeRoy Neiman, Inc.

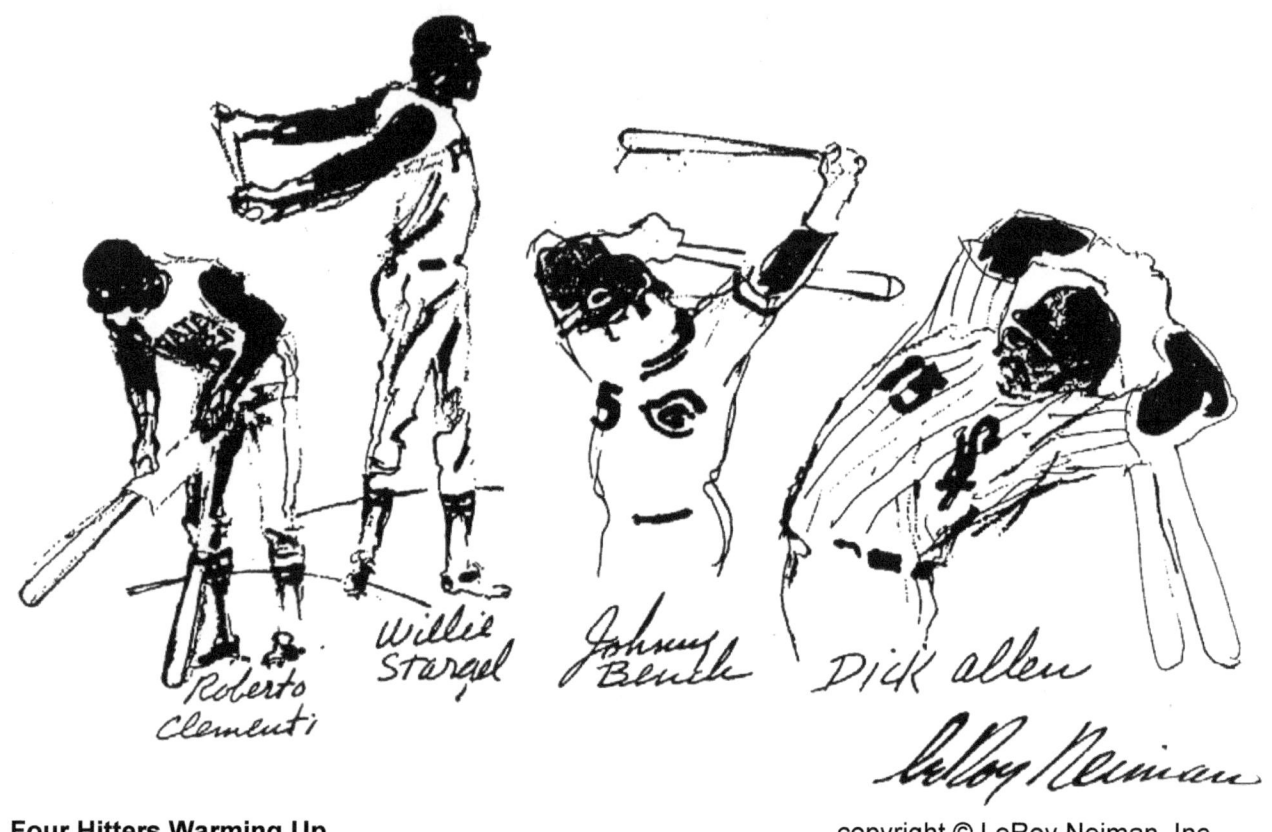

Four Hitters Warming Up   copyright © LeRoy Neiman, Inc.

Valuable baseball batting warm up exercises as taught to us by the great masters of baseball, Roberto Clemente, Willie Stargel, Johnny Bench and Dick Allen! More focused on the accessory muscles of respiration. (These diagrams together: muscles that aid breathing are being exercised in this baseball warm-up)

Physical conditioning principles for asthmatic as well as non-asthmatic people emphasize the specific components of physical fitness. For example, strength training focuses on progressive resistance exercise for specific muscle groups. Six to ten repetitions maximum are guidelines. Each muscle group is exercised for brief periods which should be within the reach of asthmatic children. Our goal is to build up progressive endurance, as tolerated, with particular emphasis on sports of the child's choice with particular breathing exercises associated with that sport.

The popularity of sports, the interest and use of their warm up exercises within the frame work of the chosen sport, and enthusiasm of sports goals keep these as interesting exercises that both children and adults look forward to doing.

All of these exercises include elbow and arm circling. Pursed lip breathing can be added to the sport exercises. Pursed lip breathing builds up a back pressure to assist and allow expiration to better and more completely empty the expired air from the chest, rather than trap air which further compresses the blocked airways.

Chest physiotherapy of staccato percussion, (repeated gentle tapping with hand in cupped position) of the chest, helps in milking and ridding the chest of mucus reinforced by postural drainage.

Running is also a stamina builder. However, short spurts of exercise of less than 4 minutes are preferred as they open or dilate the airways. Exercising at indoor gyms or health clubs until immunization of desensitization with its specific type of immunization protection in regard to the major pollen and mold season allergens are instituted.

Sports have an uplifting effect. Incorporating words of encouragement or an embracing hug also can have an uplifting effect on recovery. The excitement and enthusiasm and uplifting hugs of baseball players after winning the World Series, not to mention the time honored well televised final celebration, the 'piece de resistance' of pouring champagne over each other's head, or scoring a touchdown (all representative of outbursts of enthusiasm and cheer), as recently exemplified by Christopher Reeve when he was finally able with physical therapy to move his finger for the first time since his accident, celebrating the height of physical exercise achievement for that individual, might be utilized in sports exercises aimed towards rehabilitating the person with asthma.

FOOTBALL

Again, warm-up exercises of throwing a ball required in baseball, tennis and football.

Valuable lessons in throwing the football as taught to us by the great master of football, Joe Namath.

Stretch those muscles and enjoy watching the ball go sailing.

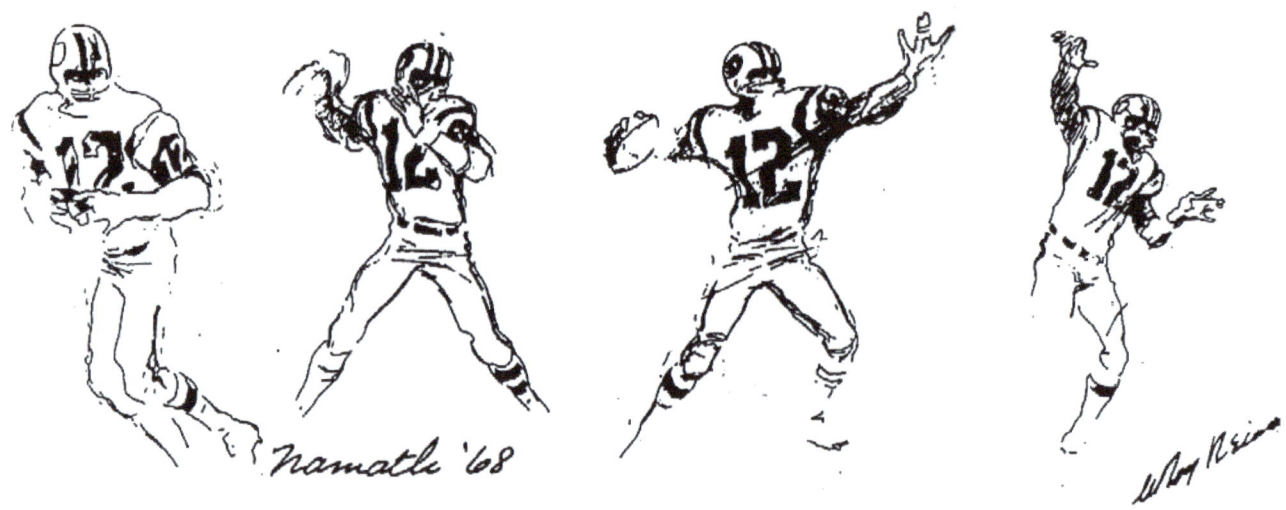

Joe Namath

copyright © LeRoy Neiman, Inc. 1968

Each throwing and catching sport, such as football shown here, helps to develop accessory muscles or respiration, so pleasant and fascinating an art to develop in a football sports exercise program.

In addition, these exercises coordinated with deep breathing and exercises to help the lymphatic circulation as well as cardiac circulation.

As we study the sports art of every sport we can visualize accessory muscles of respiration so helpfully important in a respiratory disease such as asthma.

All skills of course can be built upon more extensive encouragement, coaching (just as we cheer for our own team to win) and physical education anticipating that some of these children may indeed qualify for amateur leagues, as well as, professional. Skills are further augmented by seeking out great teachers and coaches. This bonus has not been looked upon in the past as a conceivable achievement in children with chronic respiratory diseases such as asthma. There are several examples on record of individuals who have so achieved these goals. These concepts are pioneered by Theodore Roosevelt and John. F. Kennedy, as well as, in applications of muscle disease such as Polio seen in Sister Kenney. Furthermore, I can recall several patients who have had other diseases such as trauma and if it weren't for prior physical conditioning their outcomes may not have been anywhere as successful.

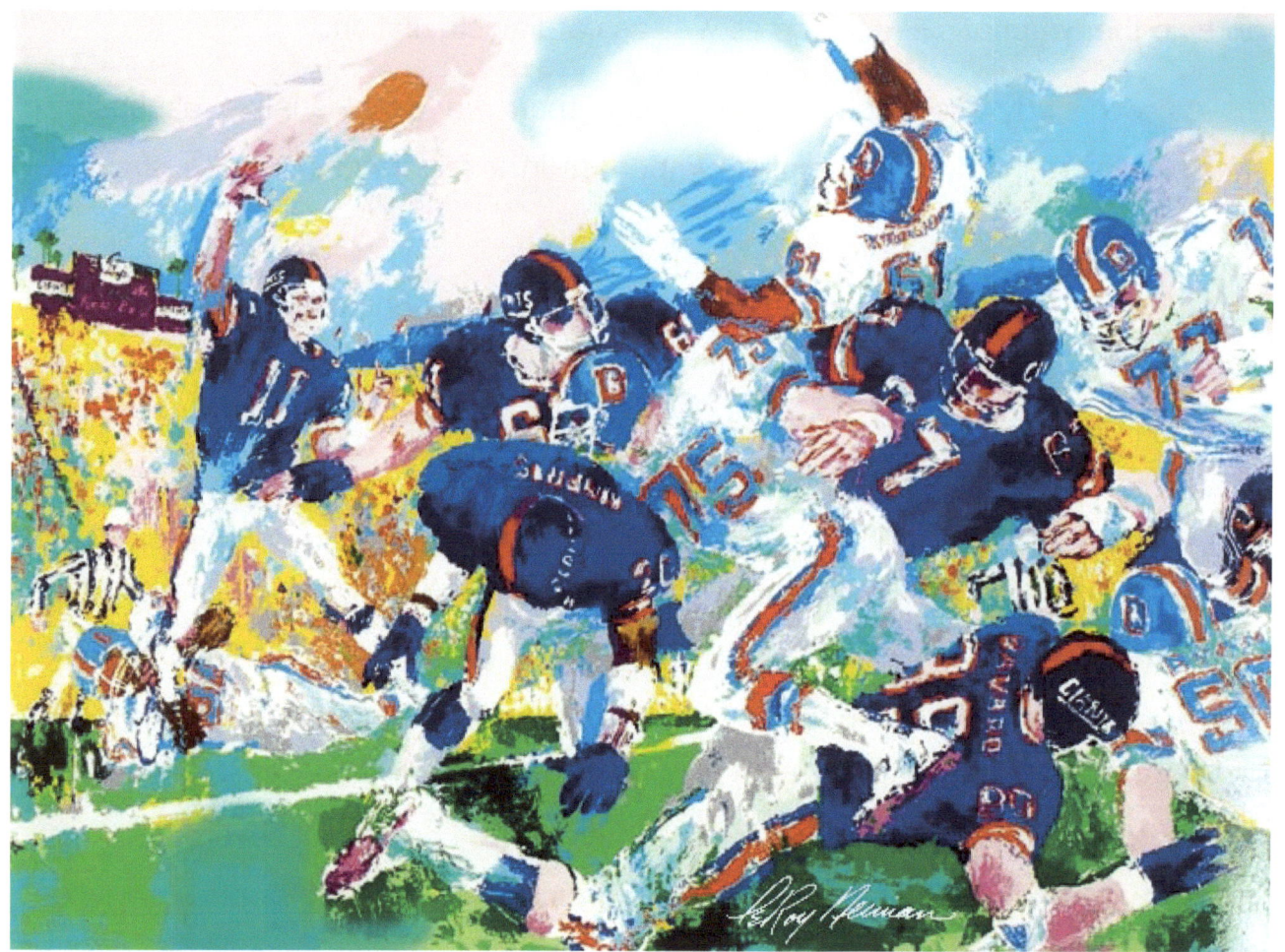

Giants – Broncos Classic

copyright © LeRoy Neiman, Inc. 1987

TENNIS

In tennis, we hold in hand a racket that is an extension of our arm incorporating swinging motions of the upper limbs. Again, we are building and conditioning as an athlete training for the Olympics, all the accessory muscles of respiration including the shoulder muscles that stabilize the chest particularly when sitting in a chair in overcoming an acute asthmatic attack, along with the chest and back muscles, along with the muscles in the neck that we can see being strained while overcoming an acute asthma attack. All with added bonuses of coordination and endurance, including the spirit of winning or achieving applied here to respiratory tract and breathing system health. In the case of a serve, the same muscles are required as football only the movements in the tennis serve are horizontal.

Throws, serves and volleys require stretching exercising and building endurance all of which use the accessory muscles of respiration.

These actions require short spurts of exercise. (Caution: regarding becoming overtired - playing a game of doubles instead of singles.)

Building general endurance allows for more efficient oxygen utilization as well as muscle development, so helpful in asthma rehabilitative exercises.

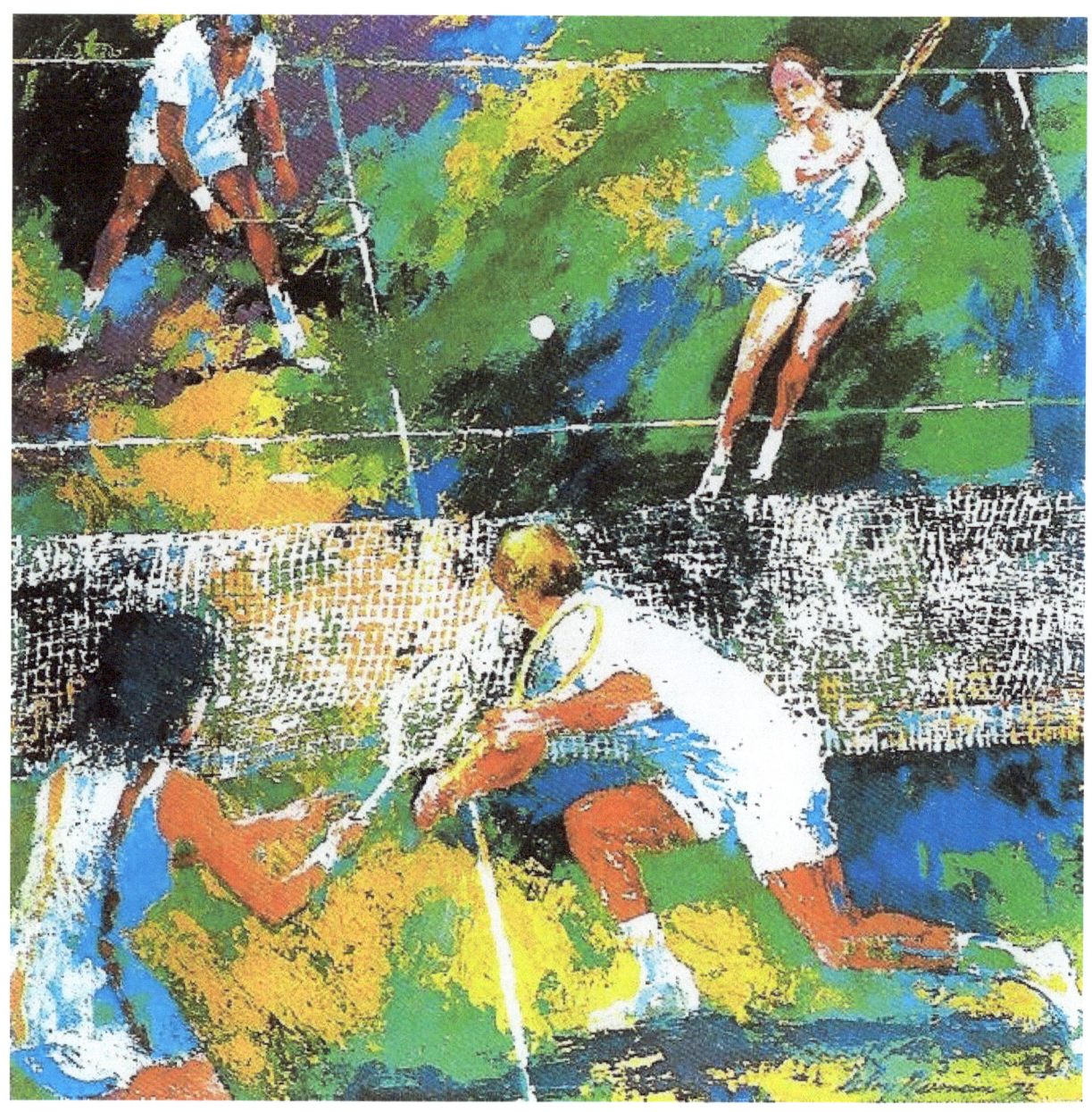

Mixed Doubles

Another great advantage of the sports philosophy is the enthusiasm for winning regardless of the odds. This feeling is a praiseworthy feeling, particularly when one is chronically ill. It is well known that stress aggravates disease and is it well known that a chronic disease is stress in itself. Anti-stress is a stimulus for recovery, it certainly is great to cheer for the home team while imbued with a sports exercise program for asthma, all applicable and appropriate to cheer one on to recovery and the goal of recovery, (additional therapeutic lessons from sports).

I saw a patient who, at age 93, was terribly sick with a very poor prognosis and it was great to see that just reaching for and putting on his baseball cap helped give him a smile despite all the adverse odds. This is an important subtle but forceful additional 'fringe benefit' feature of a sports program in medicine.

ROWING

Warm-up exercises for rowing include circling of the elbows and arms.

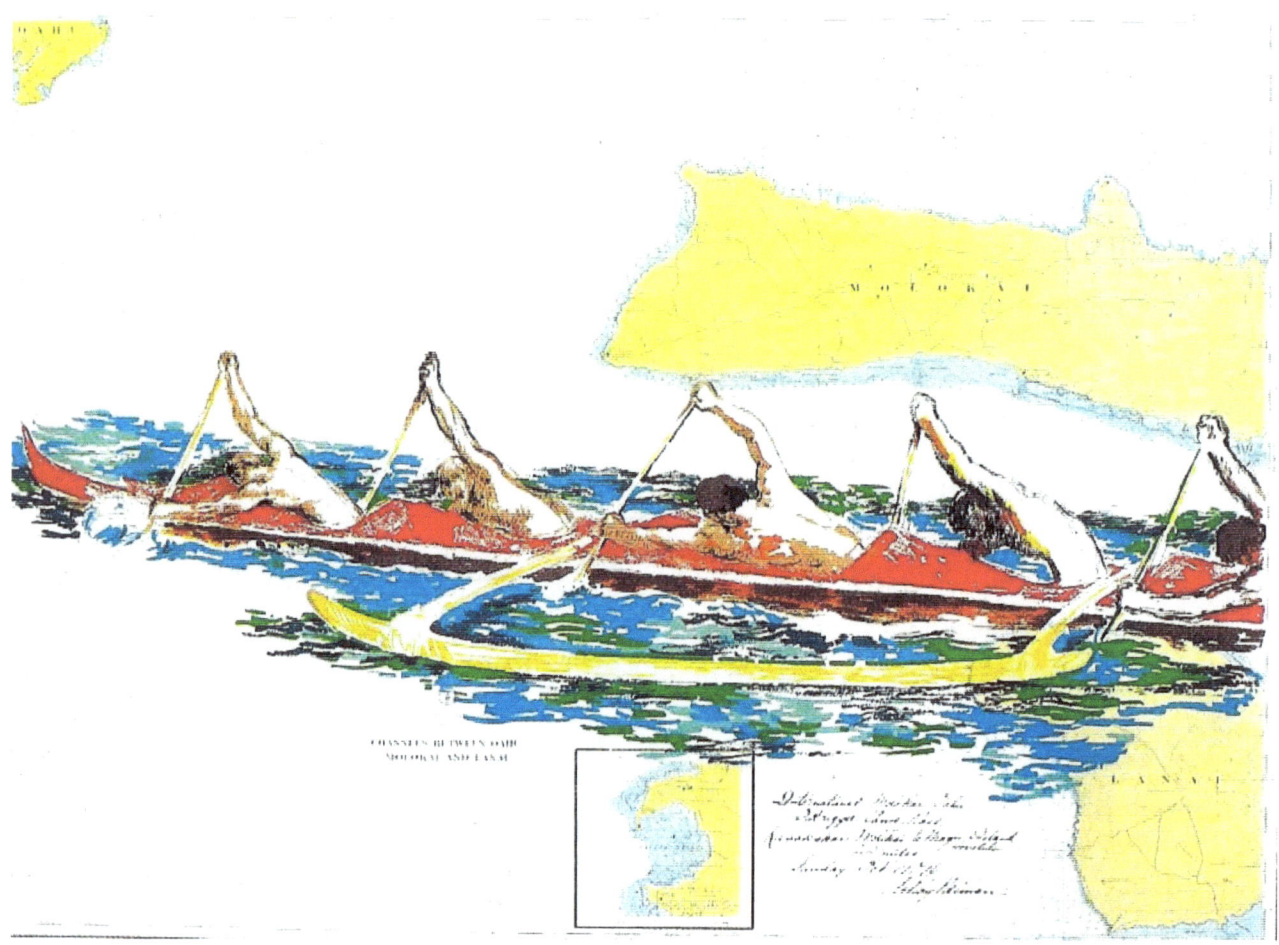

Outrigger Canoe   copyright © LeRoy Neiman, Inc. 1976

Rowing Exercises:

Rowing exercises are available in many of the apartment and condominium complexes as well as in sports exercise facilities and are even better appreciated and enjoyed when performed along with visualization of LeRoy Neiman's great sports classics paintings of rowing.

The famous paintings by Thomas Eakins, the esteemed nineteenth century Philadelphia artist of sculling (rowing) on the Schulkyll River, allows us to further appreciate even more profoundly the beautiful views that we see while driving along the Philadelphia's River Drive (or Boston's Charles River Drive). The competitive intercollegiate sport of sculling blends beautifully with the joggers, walkers and runners along the same shores.

Instituting physical and mental images of sports afford positive suggestions.

The imaging of such positive sports settings as swimming and floating on a lake or ocean along with inhaling all the clean air around the lake area, is helpful in overcoming various degrees of acute and even severe asthma.

Oral and inhaled medications are also more effective when used along with these measures of sports oriented chest physiotherapy. All performed as tolerated, wind instruments such as the recorder, harmonica, as well as humming and singing, all can be incorporated without straining with relaxation of expiration and abdominal diaphragmatic breathing. These exercises of abdominal diaphragmatic breathing can be practiced with slight pressure of book and palms of hands on the abdomen.

Normal expiration is passively dependent on the elastic recoil of the over-stretched bronchopulmonary tissue after inspiration. Various exercises can be performed which will strengthen the abdominal muscles as accessory muscles of respiration, e.g. lying on the back, raising the legs without flexing them at the knees and rotating the legs in a circular fashion. A similar abdominal muscle strengthening exercise may be performed by lying flat on one's back, followed by sitting up with arms outstretched and touching the toes and associated isometric exercises.

Also, all incorporated vibratory effects of the above measures on lower as well as upper respiratory tract and sinuses help loosen and dislodge thickened viscous mucus.

We all can enjoy a lifetime of benefit from sports respiratory exercises along with the general physical conditioning provided in this program. Not only in maximizing and rehearsing our efficacy in the CPR (cardiopulmonary resuscitation course) that we take for emergency use for our family, neighbors or co-workers, but also for ourselves as an auxiliary modality in times of respiratory illnesses.

BASKETBALL

The warm-up exercises that we have shown for baseball, football, tennis & rowing become self evident for basketball. Here, the addition of throwing a ball towards a basket is practiced. Emphasizing conditioning and coordination, in this upward projection motion of basketball and the accessory muscles of respiration the shoulders, arms, chest, back and neck muscles as we can see so beautifully depicted by the renowned sports artistry of LeRoy Neiman.

Basketball illustrated here by LeRoy Neiman incorporates the choreography of ballet and the art of hand-eye coordination in scoring. The stretching, rhythmic arching in making a basket score all accentuate the further development of the accessory muscles of respiration, so important in asthma.

The asthmatic patient envisions being able to participate in various sports, such as basketball, when his asthma is treated.

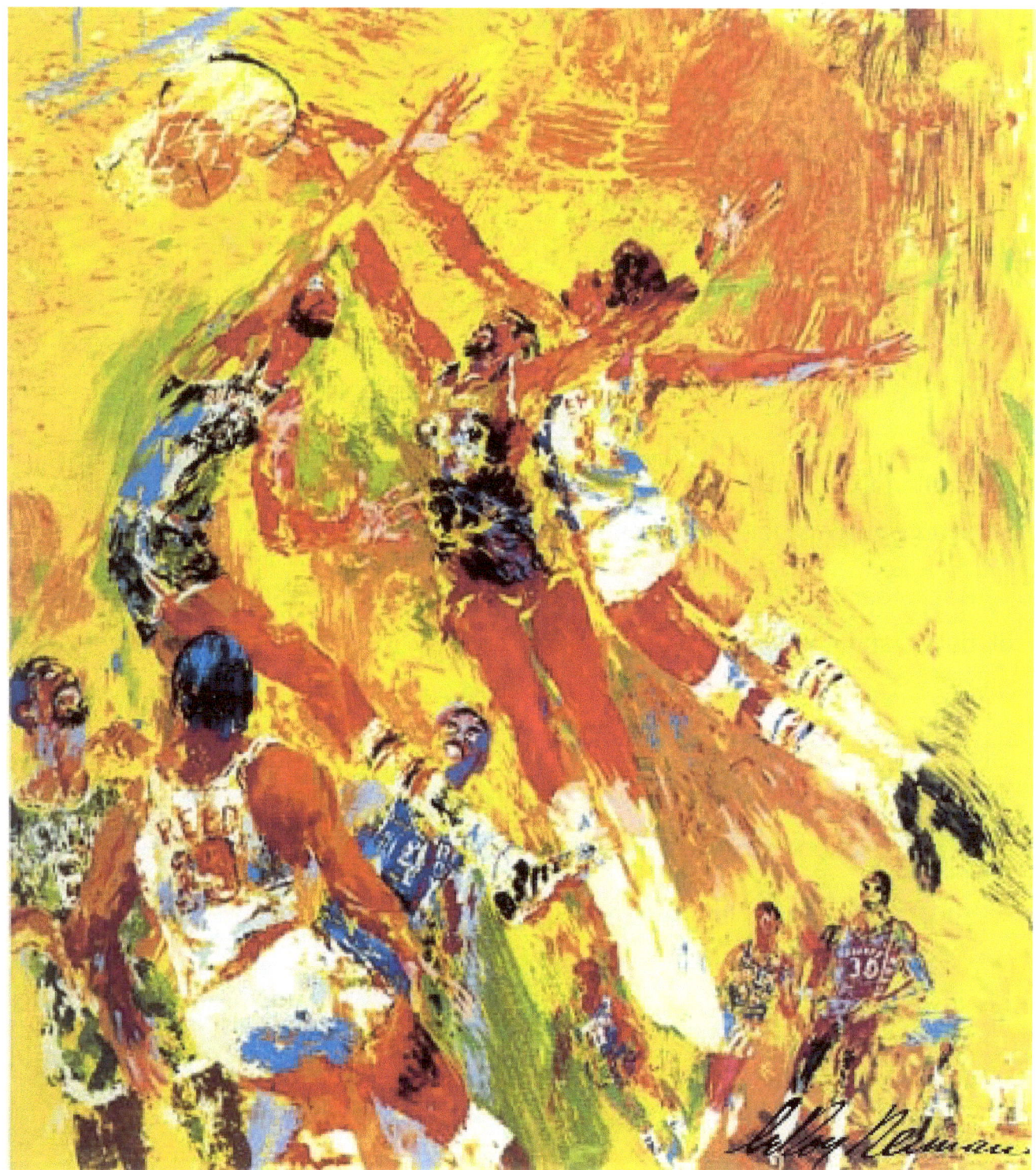

Basketball Superstars

copyright © LeRoy Neiman, Inc. 1977

JOGGING, WALKING OR RUNNING, commonly associated with all sports:

Here all warm-up exercises are accomplished through the four minute rule. The first four minutes of sports are commonly associated with production of adrenaline in the child with asthma and usually adequate to maintain an open airway during sports exercise.

Upon reaching the four minutes of continuous exercise the patient should be instructed to rest with the coach on the bench. This is the maximum opening for air exchange due to the release of adrenalin. Otherwise, the next four minutes may have adverse affects causing bronchial congestion. The patient, child and/or coach will usually pick an exercise that does not require continuous running such as baseball, or doubles as in tennis. Such sports that require running for no more than four minute increments are ideal.

Jogging, brisk walking or running should, at first be done, in the case of the asthmatic, in less than four (4) minute spurts, whether training for cross country runs or the Boston Marathon.

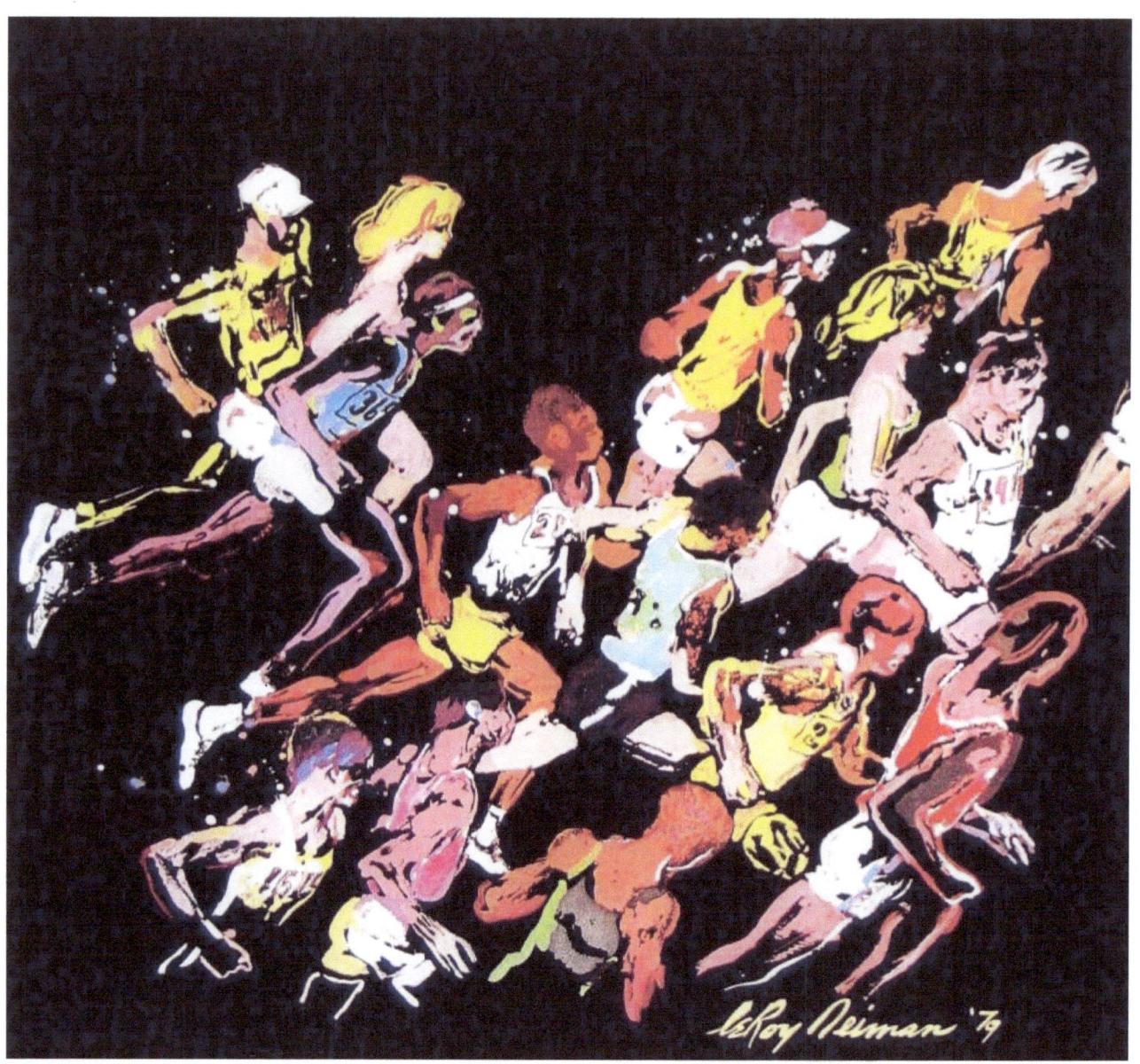

The Race, Boston Marathon   copyright © LeRoy Neiman, Inc. 1979

BALLET

The same warm-up exercises demonstrated for other sports, particularly rowing, may be practiced in ballet along with a remarkable stimulus for balanced coordination. Consider the arm and elbow circling as with such sports warm up exercises as for rowing, baseball, football, tennis along with added features of balance and coordination. Examples are presented for girls and boys in the next two figures.

Stretching and isometric exercises include using the accessory muscles of respiration as seen with the runner as he crosses the tape at the finish line and also with the breathing of an acute asthmatic. Both efforts require the support of the accessory muscles of respiration's with the asthmatic needing the additional support of holding on to the arms of a chair.

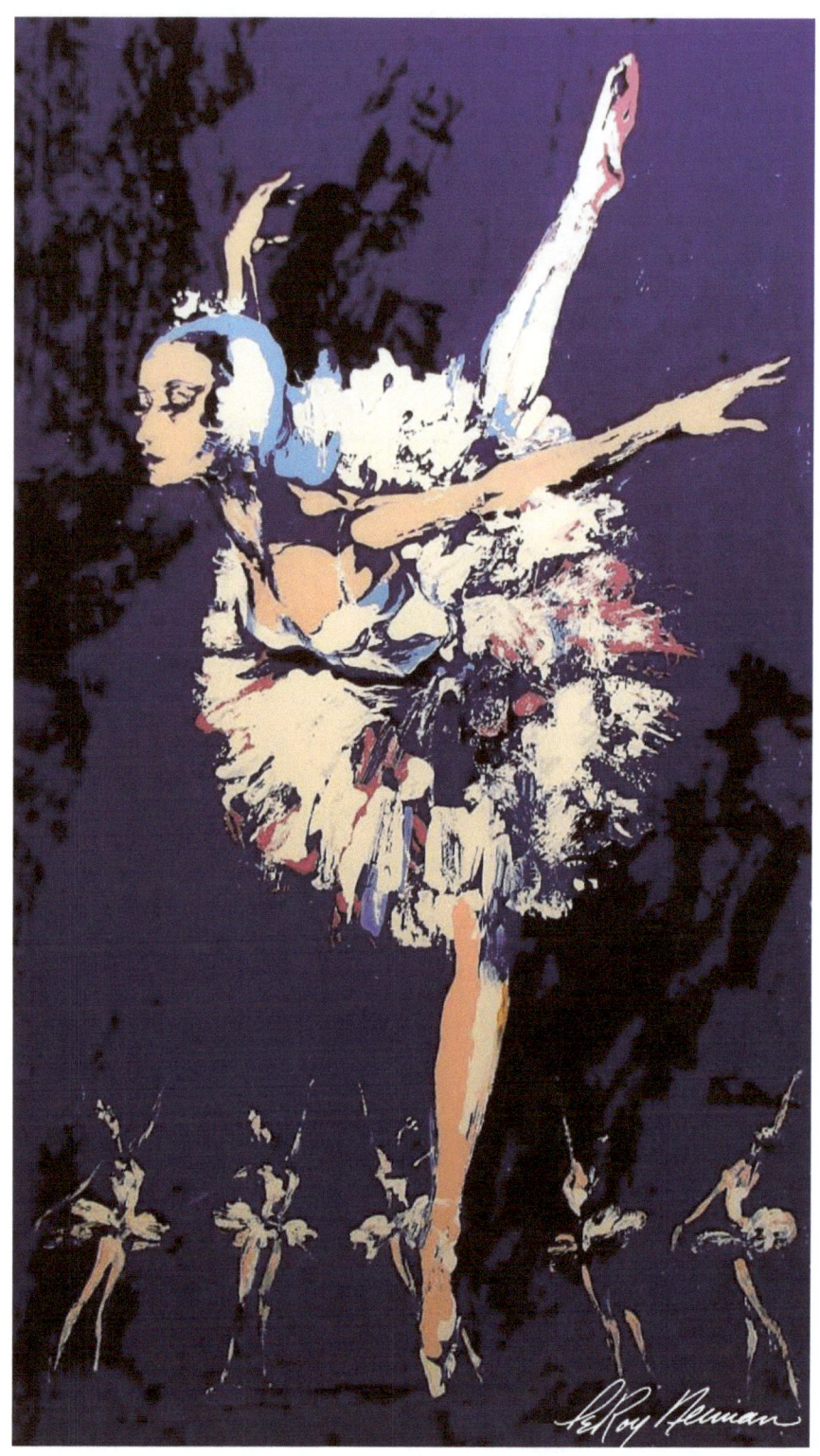

Prima Ballerina

BALLET

Imaging, isometrics, stretching and balance, skillfully and so gracefully performed in ballet, are all the while employing the accessory muscles of respiration.   Muscle control is imperative in most efficiently utilizing the accessory muscles of respiration to successfully overcome an asthmatic attack.

Paul Whiteman's observation that "asthma is rarely seen in a windy instrument player" probably extends to sports.

These accessory muscles being trained to best achieve in most sports, such as the runner crossing the finish line at a track meet, where similar accessory muscles of respiration are used, just as they are used during an acute asthmatic attack.

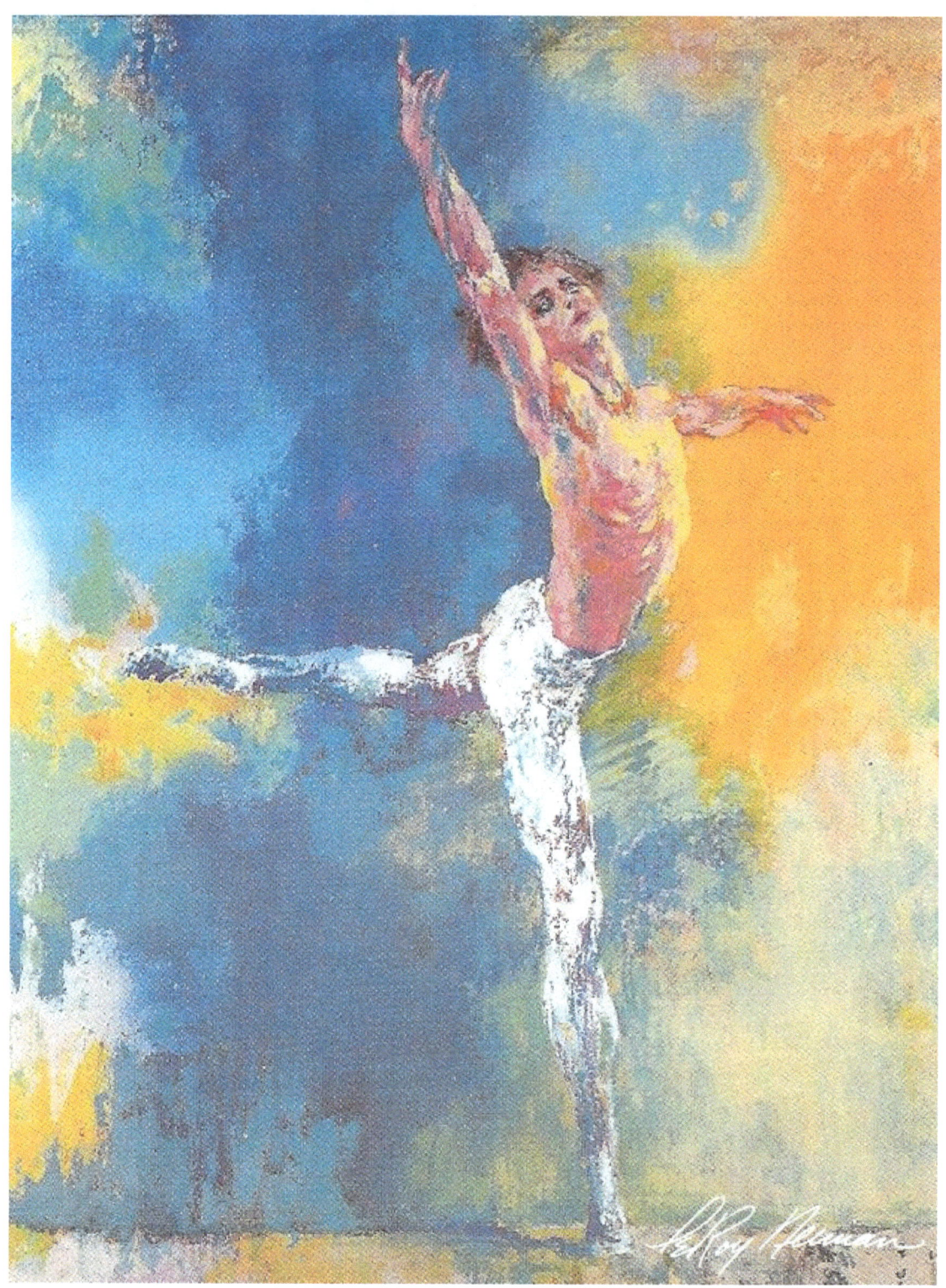

Mikhail Baryshnikov

copyright © LeRoy Neiman, Inc. 1983

SKIING

One caution for some asthmatic patients associated with skiing are the blasts of cold air functioning as a bronchial irritant. If we can eliminate inhalation of cold air these exercises may also be profoundly helpful. An alternative solution is the use of indoor elliptical machines, which mimic the motions of outdoor skiing. It is important to remember that the four minute of sports exercise followed by brief rest rule, always applies no matter what sport or exercise is performed.

Warm up exercises for skiing help develop accessory muscles of respiration, along with the added feature of development of coordination and agility, lost with chronic illness such as asthma.

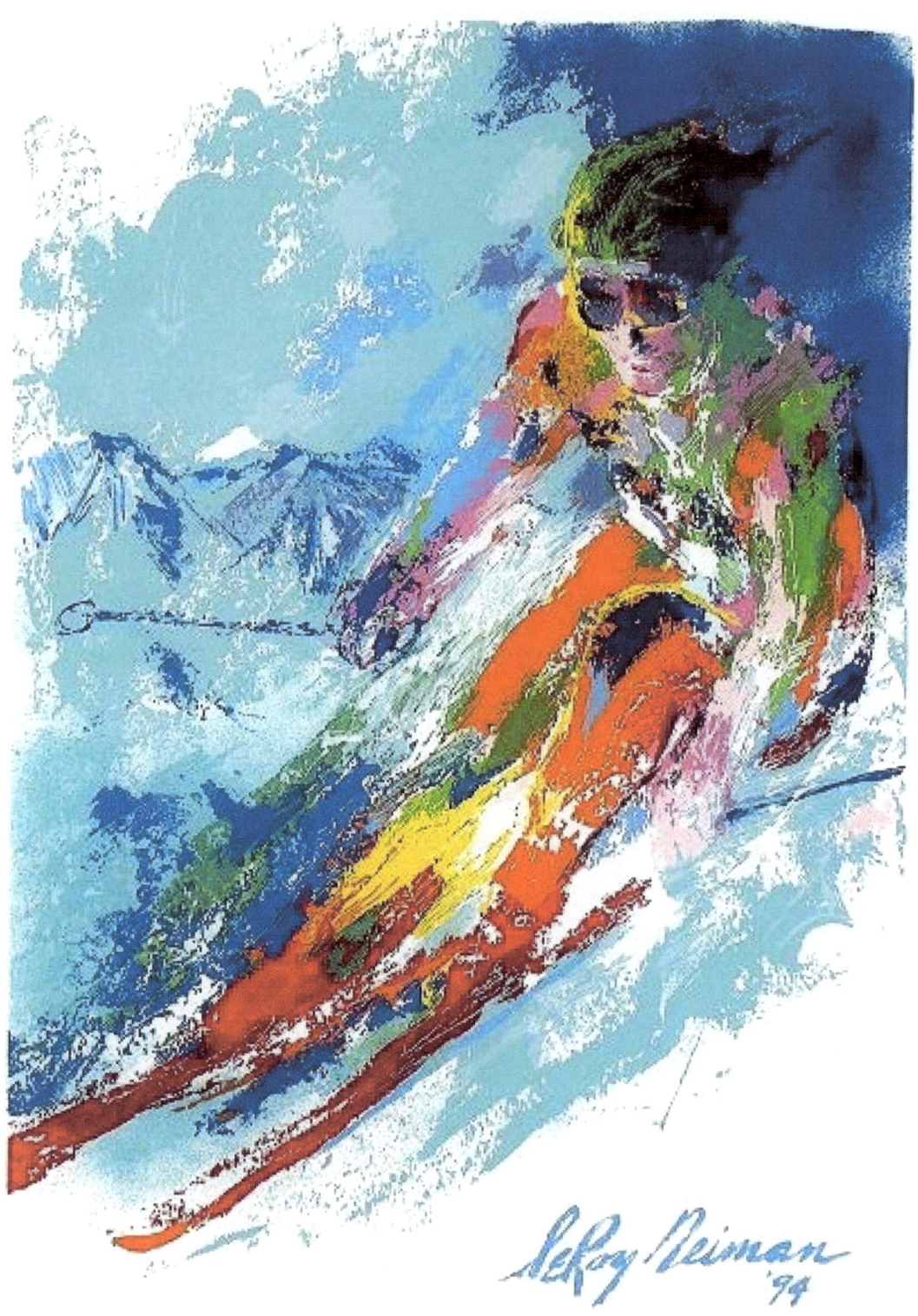

World Class Skier

SOCCER

In soccer, the warm-up exercises are excellent, but both the child and coach must keep in mind the four minute rule when participating. This is followed by the reward of a brief rest on the bench, necessary in order to prevent bronchial congestion. Outdoor sports such as soccer, baseball & football should be looked upon with caution due to the exposure of allergens (i.e. pollen, mold, dust). Watering down the fields may serve as preventative factor in further irritating the child's airways.

Ideally, indoor sports, such as tennis, basketball and dance, would have this advantage of environmental control by using air conditioning. Moreover, playing tennis doubles would also be an advantage because of the interruptions and rest periods, which obey the four minute rule. Coach's of other sports can do the same by breaking up playing time and enhancing the most tolerable. This strategy of sports superimposed on the strategies of sports, asthma and exercise are very useful in sports exercise conditioning.

Warm up exercises for soccer help develop the accessory muscles of respiration, along with the added feature of development of coordination and agility, frequently lost with chronic illness such as asthma.

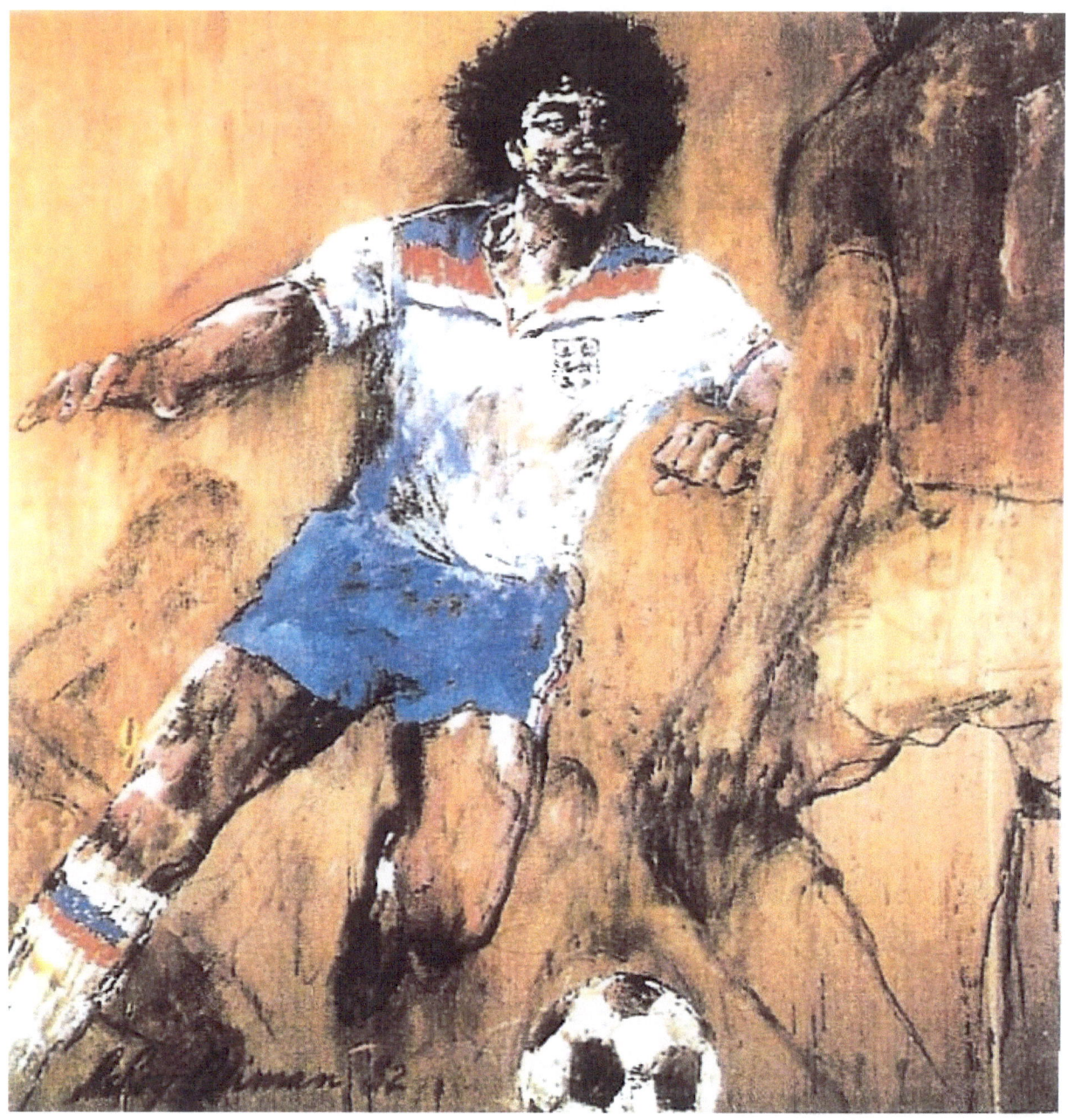

Kevin Keegan

A brief overview of breathing normally and without difficulty

The purpose of breathing is to provide oxygen for cell function and to remove carbon dioxide which is a waste product of cell function. In general there are processes of external transfer of the air we breathe into our lungs, followed by internal transfer of oxygen and carbon dioxide to all tissues.

The problem for an asthmatic is difficulty in getting air both in and out. This is true but especially so when the child or adult becomes allergic to something, such as pollen, mold, cat or dog. The air in their lungs becomes "trapped" so there is no space for the "fresh" air to get into or out of their lungs. Some of this "entrapment" is caused by the fluids and swelling that build up due to the allergic reaction. This leads us to the therapeutic procedures described in the following sections. The internal process at the cell level is improved when external breathing makes more oxygen available (air in) and sends more carbon dioxide out (air out).

BREATHING EXERCISES

Breathing exercises are helpful in overcoming broncho-spasm, and increasing the function of the accessory muscles of respiration. Slow expiration through pursed lips, as if gently blowing a bugle, is a most effective breathing exercise.

PURSED LIP BREATHING

Here, the children, young adults and family members can be inspired by band leaders such as Paul Whiteman who have noted the benefits of playing wind instruments on health in preventing health conditions such as asthma.

Pursed Lip Breathing

Wind instruments serving as another very pleasant breathing exercise

A study performed with as prominent leader of the "big bands" revealed that band members playing wind instruments were much less likely to develop asthma than the rest of the band. The bandleader, Paul Whiteman, has been cited at the National Allergy Meetings as one of the bandleaders involved.

LeRoy Neiman may be congratulated on advancing what might be looked upon as *modern impressionistic art*.

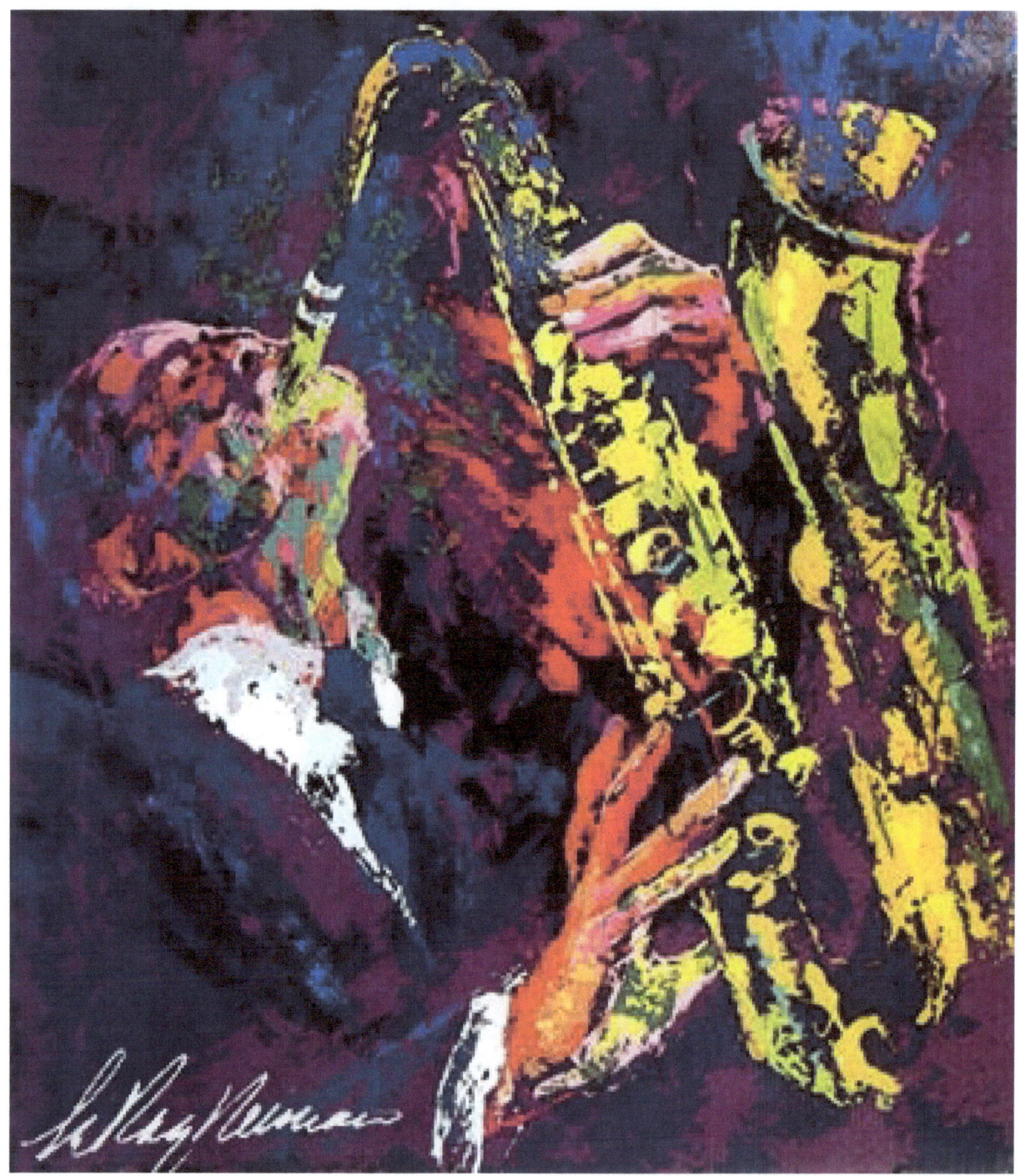

Saxman

The physiologic principles and mechanism of pursed lip breathing:

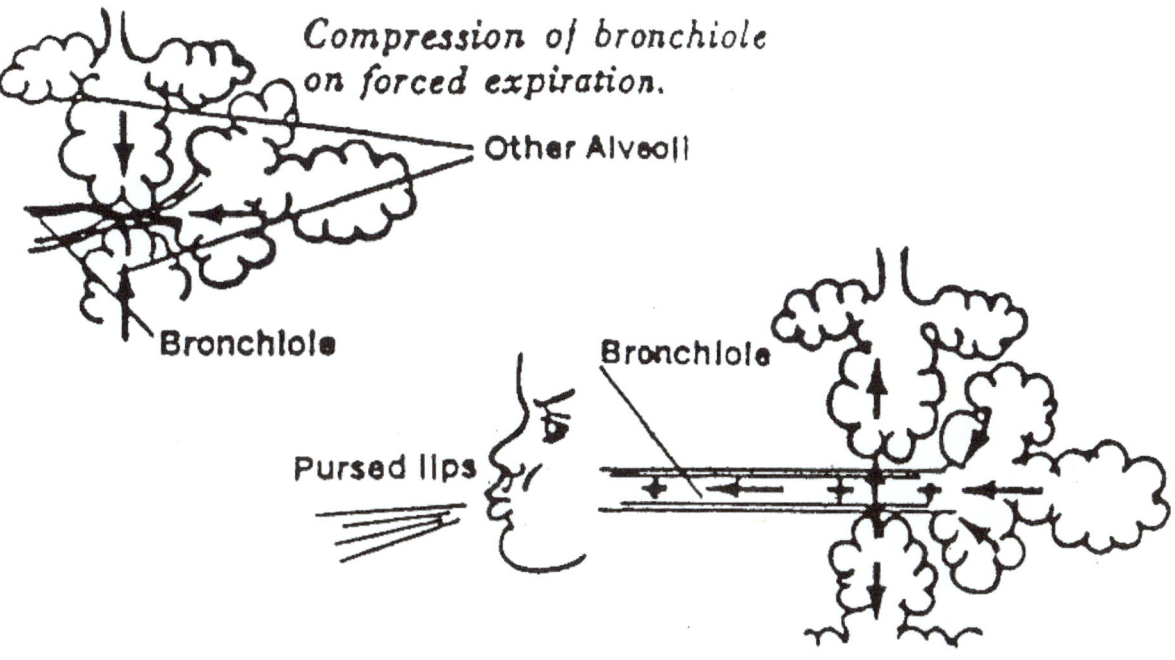

Compression of bronchiole on forced expiration.

Other Alveoli

Bronchiole

Pursed lips

Bronchiole

Pursed lip breathing by creating positive pressure lengthens expiration and prevents collapse of bronchioles.

The physiologic principles of pursed lip breathing:

The mechanics of pursed lip breathing help in overcoming "dynamic airway obstruction" magnified by expiratory collapse of the bronchi occurring with exertion. The breathing with and after exertion, exercise or emotional disturbance such as crying is not only forceful but also rapid hyperventilation which causes more expiratory collapse, dyspnea and starts a vicious cycle. The pursed lip breathing exercise therefore is taught to be combined with slow relaxed breathing.

A study performed with a prominent leader of the "big bands" revealed that band members playing wind instruments were much less likely to develop asthma than the rest of the band. Paul Whiteman has been cited at the National Allergy Meetings as one of the bandleaders involved. With practice, the patient can be taught to use this breathing pattern in place of rapid panicky breathing, seen in some patients with acute bronchial asthma.

Shoulder girdle exercises such as swinging or rotating the arms in a windmill-like manner or moving the arms and elbows in a rowing motion (elbow circling) can easily be mastered by children and adults. Also, the asthmatic person may be taught to breathe more deeply by using their abdominal muscles. It has been observed that asthmatic children instinctively breathe with their abdominal muscles.

Abdominal breathing with contraction of the abdominal muscles on expiration may be regarded as an added pump and active form of respiration, as opposed to the natural or passive breathing on expiration of the normal person.

PURSED LIP BREATHING

The memory trick or 'mnemonic' to remember the helpful affect of pursed lip breathing is to breathe with pursed lips onto the palm of your hand. The blown air should feel cool, not hot when pursed lip breathing is performed properly.

Pursed Lip Breathing

1. Breathe out slowly. You should be making soft blowing sound if done properly, breath should feel cool.

2. Keep up and maintain breathing out as long as you can, at least twice as long as you take to breathe in.

3. It may help to use a timer (metronome) allowing, for example, three half-second beats for breathing in and six beats for breathing out.

4. Pursed lip breathing can be practiced by blowing a paper, wisp of cotton, Kleenex or ping pong ball across the table.

Pursed Lip Breathing

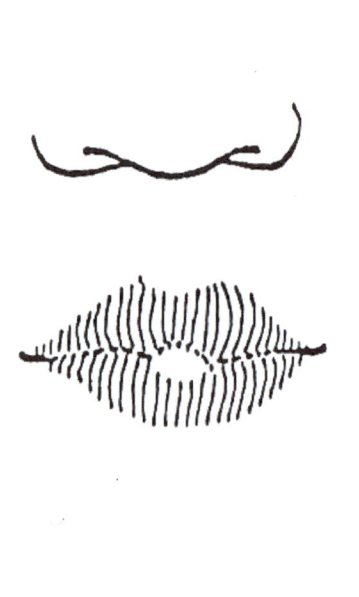

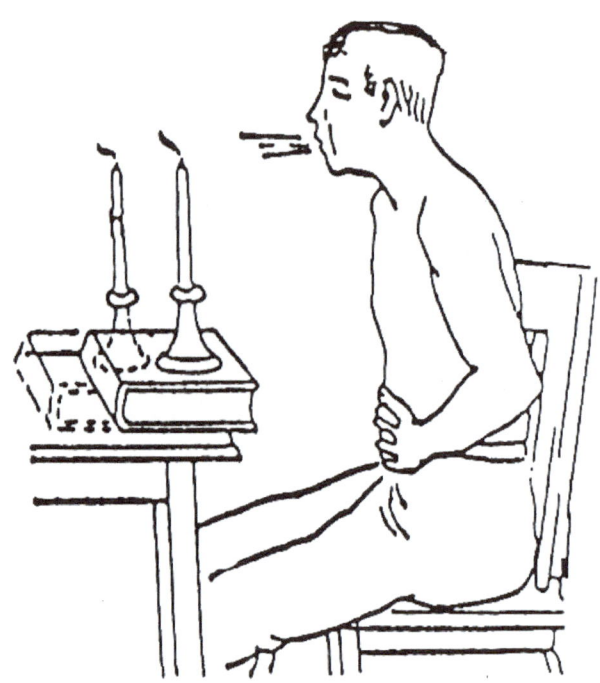

Breathing Exercises of Chest Physiotherapy

The purpose of the breathing exercises of chest physiotherapy is to drain the tracheobronchial air passages of excess mucus in asthma and allergic bronchitis. Breathing exercises repeated after asthma medication or inhaled asthma medication would further rid the airway of trapped mucus and also trapped air. Further prescribed dosages of inhalant medication will be impelled onto the mucous membrane rather than onto the mucus.

Chest Physiotherapy

Gentle chest pounding (with the important <u>element of gentleness</u>) or percussion with cupped hand as well as vibratory physical therapy over the chest also helps to loosen mucus.

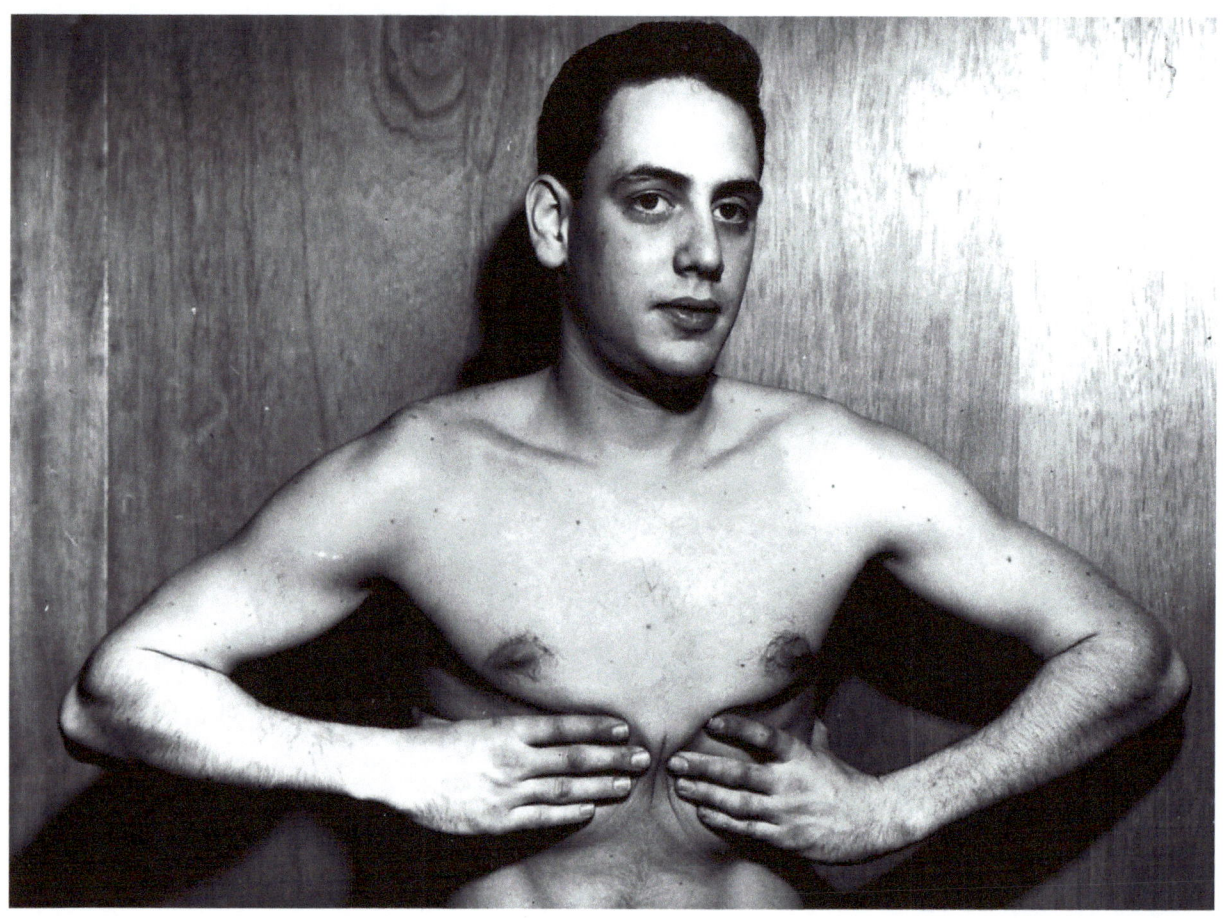

Finally, a method of squeezing this very viscous gelatinous mucus from the tracheobronchial tube is utilized shortly after bronchodilator therapy. The patient with staccato expiration, through pursed lips, squeezes the chest with his hands in an effort to expel or milk the mucus from the tracheo- bronchial tree.

Drainage of Mucus

Postural drainage may prove helpful to persons with excessive mucus. They should be instructed to lie on the bed, abdomen down, with the head and upper portion of the body (chest) hanging over the edge of the bed (as if searching for a shoe).

Drainage of Mucus

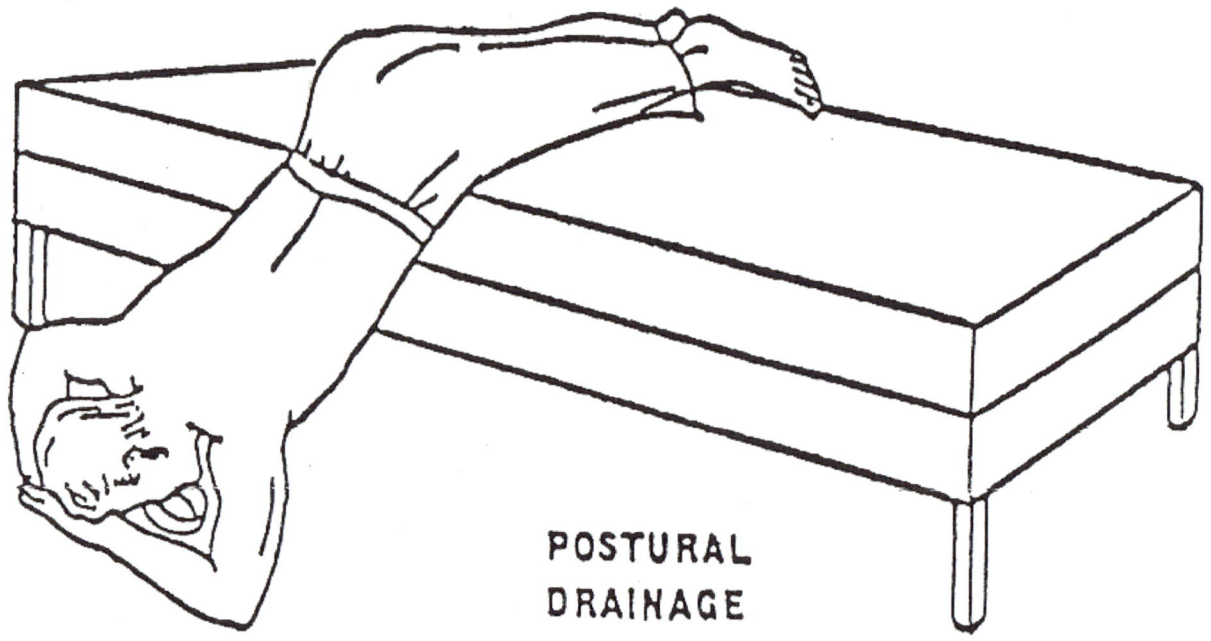

POSTURAL
DRAINAGE

Drainage of Mucus

Working together through sports warm up and breathing exercises we have developed accessory muscles of respiration in conjunction with increased coordination and also incorporated the four minute rule and pursed lip breathing to keep airways open.

Now we further use different measures to milk the chest of small plugs of mucus (shown in these next photographs).

Dr. Laennec, the chest physician who in the mid 1800's invented the stethoscope, an invention that was inspired by watching two children transmit a message by scratching a pin on a wooden plank see-saw, also discovered these small plugs of obstructive asthmatic mucus and named them tapioca-like pearls.

These obstructive lumps of mucus coughed up in asthma are referred to as the pearls of Dr. Laennec, acknowledging his discovery. The next two photos exemplify the drainage by a cupping action associated with postural drainage. The back is on both right and left sides. This may be simulated by the action of turning the patient over "like a pancake until they are well done!"

Steps Incorporated With Postural Drainage Of Mucus

In a child, postural drainage may be accomplished by laying the child in the trough-like space of the outstretched legs and adding cupped hand percussion over all the surfaces of the chest.

The child may be rotated to both lateral obliques, both anterior and posterior positions.

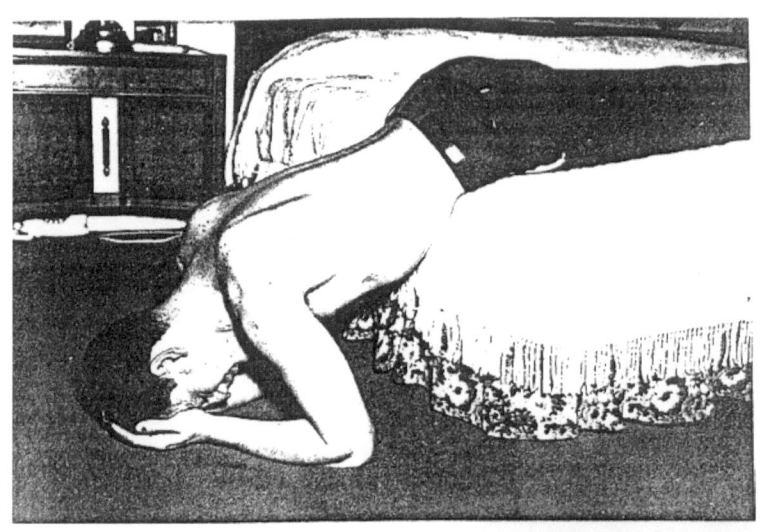

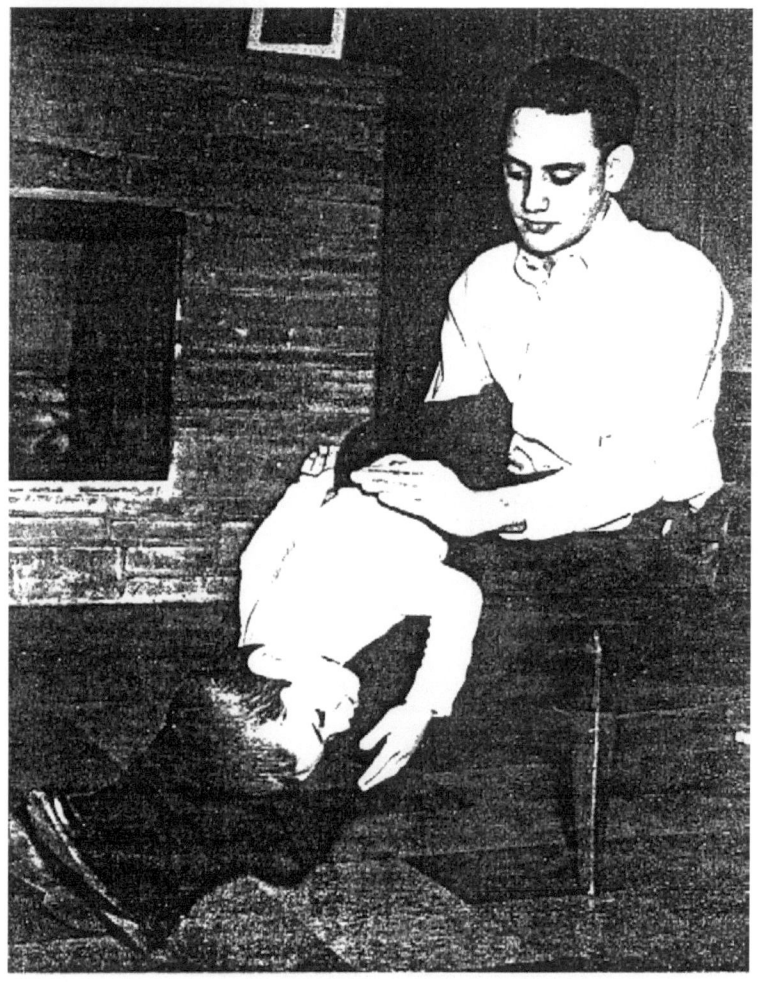

Postural Drainage

Postural drainage should be done before meals and before retiring at night. While in this position the following exercises should be done also:

Postural drainage of mucus in a child may be accomplished by laying the child in the trough-like space of the parent's outstretched legs and adding cupped hand percussion over all surfaces of the chest.

The child may be rotated to both lateral oblique, anterior and posterior positions for the gentle percussion action.

Chest Breathing Exercises – review

1. Cupped hand percussion of chest.

2. Vibrating staccato motion at end of expiration and general massage of the chest and back.

3. Lie face down across the bed with head and upper part of the body extending over the side of the bed. For adults, from hips down stays on the bed. Let upper part of the body bend downward so that you can rest your head on your hands against the floor.

4. While face down, cough in a series of gentle "throat-clearing" coughs, holding your breath for a moment after each one and then breathing in gently. This is to bring out any mucus that has drained from deep down in your lungs into the larger air passages.

5. While in this position, it is helpful to have a family member use gentle cupped hand percussion followed by staccato vibratory motion, also performed gently, alternately on the back and front of the chest, then on the sides, as tolerated. This aids in postural drainage of mucus.

    For a small child, to perform the above type of exercise, carefully hold the child in an out-stretched position, in a similar inverted fashion, on the legs of the parent whose legs are acting as a trough for support. These steps all help to rid the person of impacted mucus.

6. Fluids, (including warm dilute tea with plenty of lemon or lime) and several glasses of water daily will help to thin mucus and make its production easier to expel.

How To Cough Usefully

Coughing serves a very useful purpose. This means careful controlled coughs.

The philosophy here is to treat each person gently. Hard coughing may do harm. The blast of air jetting out of your lung tubes and windpipe can get rid of unwanted blocks in the passages, including excess and thick mucus (phlegm).

Those plugs of mucus were first described by Laennec, a famous French chest physician who invented the stethoscope, as pearls of Laennec. This mucus is vividly described as pearls of tapioca-like white mucus. If the mucus is discolored, yellowish or green, a respiratory infection should be suspected and treated accordingly. Doing so will prevent unnecessary asthma flare ups.

You can make your cough more useful in getting rid of mucus in this way:

1. While sitting down, clasp your arms across your abdomen.

2. As you cough, press clasped hands in against your abdomen. This will add force to the jet of air coming out of your lungs.

3. Before you start to cough, get as much air in your lungs as possible.

4. Keep your head forward. Hold your breath for a moment after each cough, then breathe in gently, to keep from sucking the phlegm back in.

Special Breathing Exercises

Arm and Elbow circling

DO EXERCISES <u>TWICE</u> <u>DAILY</u>

Additional Methods to Improve Breathing

1. Swimming (just make sure to dry hair thoroughly, especially in winter months).

2. Musical (wind) instruments, e.g., harmonica, flute-like instruments

3. Another extension of breathing exercises is singing with relaxed breathing. All of the breathing apparatus is used as in relaxed breathing exercise fashion taught here. Proper singing or speaking can be carried out effectively by taking in relatively small amounts of air. The spoken or singing voice should then be projected breathing out in relaxed fashion. The pursed lip breathing and abdominal and accessory muscles of respiratory breathing can be practiced while taking a walk.

This is the method that Demosthenes, the famous Greek orator, used while walking along the seashore, to practice being heard above the sound of the waves. (Microphones, of course, were not available then).

We have also encouraged incorporating sports warm up exercises in developing accessory muscles of respiration along with gymnastics at school and at home.

A new meaning to the choreography of physical education

'Gotta dance' Gene Kelly, 'everyone can dance.' The rhythmic movement of walking is a form of dancing. Walking is now considered to be the most common rediscovered and emphasized form of conditioning as applied to heart disease

In addition, these exercises coordinated with deep breathing and breathing exercises help the lymphatic circulation as well as cardiac circulation

At the same time highly motivational fitting in muscles are respiration and their accessory muscles to the rhythmic dance dedicated to a high level of efficiency of performance of professional sports.

Concurrent with conditioning for enhanced fitness and respiratory fitness to enhance oxygenation in asthma, the individual with asthma through this physical conditioning program also has now acquired advanced physical fitness and respiratory fitness for the acute asthmatic attack.

In a sense, he has used the techniques of the professional athlete in training for a tournament in conjunction with specially adapted warm up exercises and chest physiotherapy to accomplish his much needed physical fitness goals.

For a child with asthma, just as this illness has gotten him behind in school subjects such as math or English, this program allows him to catch up on physical fitness and physical education in sports so he can be equal to and in some cases, ahead of his peers. This is equally important in every way for the adult.

A new meaning to the choreography of physical education "Gotta dance," Gene Kelly's noted comment almost everyone can dance using the same rhythmic movement as in walking which is a form of dance.

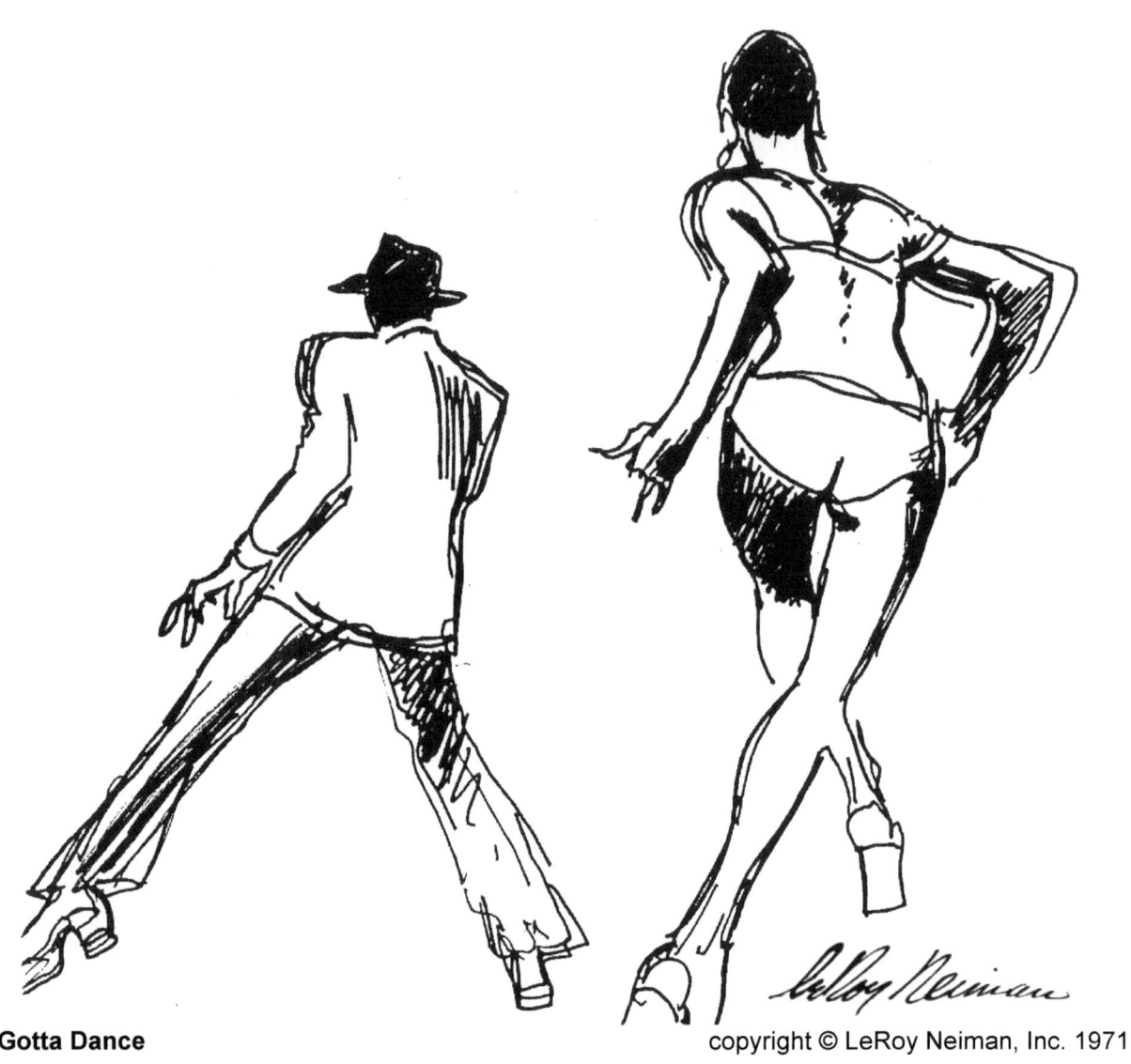

Gotta Dance

WALKING

Walking is the most common re-discovered sport wherein form and conditioning, as in dancing, can be emphasized. Walking is also a current exercise application in heart disease.

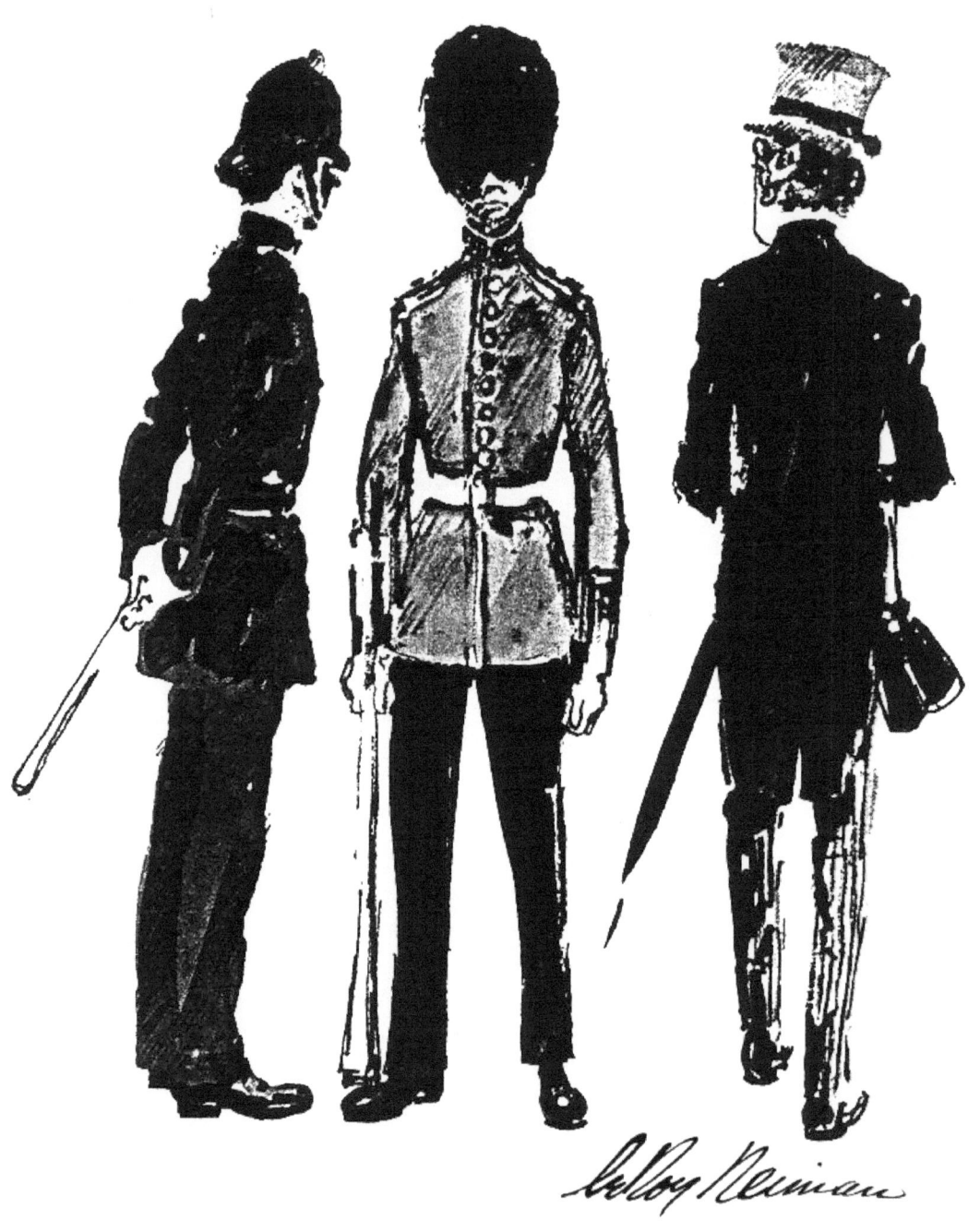

The British Male

copyright © LeRoy Neiman, Inc. 1972

Motivationally appropriate is the enhancement of conditioning and development of muscles used in respiration and their accessory muscles to the rhythmic dance dedicated to a high level of efficiency of performance in sports.

Concurrent with conditioning for enhanced fitness and respiratory fitness is the need of oxygenation in asthma. The individual with asthma also requires physical fitness and respiratory fitness to help himself or herself during an acute asthmatic attack. He or she unknowingly uses the techniques of the athlete training for a tournament.

Where else in life do we find such outbursts of encouraging enthusiasm as in sports? It is this encouraging vision that we found has made this sports exercise program so exciting to children as well as adults.

SUMMARY:

Chest physiotherapy in conjunction with prescribed sports warm up exercises:

1. In allergic asthma selected aspects of a sport are prescribed to build general stamina and strengthen muscles of respiration. Do not do exercise to the point of symptoms or fatigue. Indoor sports such as basketball may have an advantage in allergic disease, with indoor courts at school, the gym or at the 'Y'.

2. Exercise, if possible with the least mold and/or pollen exposure. The peak of noonday sun minimizes pollution, mold and pollen exposure. In a sense, the noonday sun breaks through the pollution inversion.

3. Sports warm up exercises that the asthmatic would find appealing as well as useful during treatment.

4. Sports the asthmatic patient envisions being able to do when his asthma is treated and under good control.

5. Short spurt exercises of less than 4 minutes such as ball chasing helps keep the airway open.

Caution: Continuous exercise, (more than 4 minutes) such as with soccer or basketball only if excellent progress and condition permits as it may worsen broncho-spasm and asthma.

6. Enhancing skills, efficacy and coordination of chest muscular pumping through sports warm-up exercises.

7. Further helping this pumping action, the four minute rule when adrenaline output is favorable in 'guiding the coach' and child regarding the time limit to rest when major exertion is required, (i.e. four minute mile). This tolerated exercise time limit may be extended with progressive conditioning in conjunction with allergy care, pursed lip breathing, postural drainage and companion breathing exercises. With regard to pursed lip breathing, double check to make sure cool air is blown out (by blowing through pursed lip upon the palm test).

All About Allergies & Asthma

Although allergies and asthma affect over 50 and 34 million Americans respectively, they are among the most misunderstood and misdiagnosed of all chronic ailments.

Symptoms which may go unrecognized include nasal congestion (often misdiagnosed as a stubborn cold or sinus problem); upset stomach (frequently blamed on emotional tension); and dry, itchy skin (sometimes regarded as dermatitis due to nerves). No wonder allergies are known in medical circles as "Little imitators."

An allergy can be defined as a case of mistaken identity in which an individual's overly protective immune system attacks a substance which is totally harmless in most other people.

Allergic symptoms, however, frequently do not develop on first contact. The body requires a certain amount of exposure to the allergen, or irritating substance, in order to develop this hypersensitivity which is caused by the harmful antibodies known as Immunoglobulin E (IgE).

Respiratory Allergies

Let's say a child is prone to hay fever – a common allergy to the pollen of trees, grass and weeds. The first time this child inhales the offending pollen his immune system swings into action and begins to produce the damaging IgE antibodies.

It takes about three months of exposure to pollen for the respiratory system to get the message, become sensitized and prepare to fight back.

Since ragweed season in this part of the country only lasts about six weeks per year, the child will not develop symptoms until he is at least three years old. From then on, every time the youngster inhales the offending pollen, the special sensitized cells in his respiratory tract will release granules of histamines causing allergic symptoms of congestion and swelling of the mucous membranes. These symptoms are nature's way of localizing or "walling off" the suspected invader.

The most important hay fever season in the Northeast begins around August 15th. Anyone who develops a lingering, late summer cold should seriously consider the possibility of hay fever. If untreated, it can render an individual susceptible to asthma, a more serious congestive allergic problem contributing to almost 4,000 deaths annually.

Seasonal Allergies (Spring – tree pollens, Summer – grass pollens, and Fall – weed pollens, best examples ragweed)

Other pollen allergies from trees and grass develop in the spring, when mild temperatures cause the production and release of these pollens.

In all types of pollen allergy, the patient usually feels better on rainy days because the rain washes the pollen out of the air. These patients feel worse during early morning hours when most pollen is shed.

Two other irritating, warm weather inhalants probably more devastating than pollen are atmospheric mold and mildew, which grows outdoors on dead leaves and wet grass. Indoors, a damp basement, an unvented clothes dryer, even many houseplants are common breeding grounds. Mold and mildew can produce nasal congestion and even asthma in allergic individuals.

Contact Dermatitis

Another type of allergic reaction known as contact dermatitis involves poison ivy. The culprit here is an oily substance known as urushiol which is present on the leaves of poison ivy, poison oak and poison sumac. When an allergic individual comes in contact with any of these plants, a special component of his white cells sounds the alarm in the skin tissues. The result is the itchy, blistering rash which develops at the point of contact.

Many people mistakenly believe that a poison ivy rash can be spread by scratching the blisters. Actually, it is not the fluid inside the blisters which perpetuates the rash, but the remaining oily substance which is spread around the skin by scratching. To prevent this from happening, use hydrogen peroxide which helps deactivate the allergen. Contaminated clothing and shoes, of course should be thoroughly cleaned.

Treatment

Symptoms of many mild forms of allergy can be controlled by avoidance of the irritating substance, although the use of antihistamines and decongestants may be required.

Symptoms of more severe allergies can be reduced, or even eliminated, with a series of desensitizing injections against those substances not readily avoidable.

Sports exercise includes the following three levels to the management of allergies and asthma:

1. The avoidance of offending allergens wherever practicable.
2. Improvement of the patient's tolerance to allergens by desensitization with specific allergens.
3. Use of temporary measures which include symptomatic anti-allergic drug therapy.

The object of allergy care is to reduce the allergic load, where possible, by avoidance.

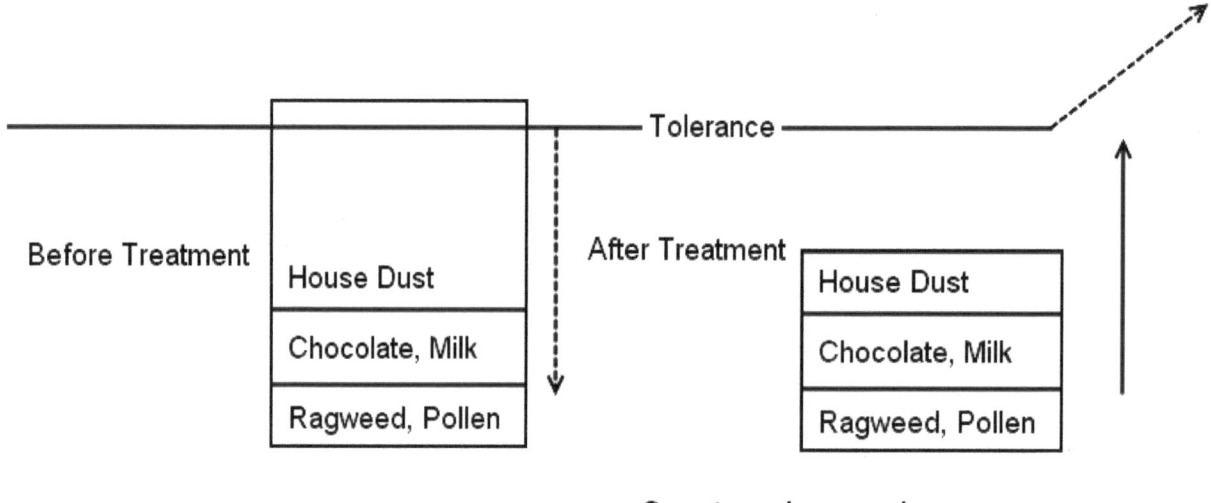

General health measures, e.g. adequate exercise, nutrition, rest and avoidance of specific allergens where possible, e.g. avoidance or minimizing house dust, the simplest method is directed to the bedroom, to reduce the allergic asthmatic disease load (these principles hold true in management of any disease).

To improve resistance to the allergic asthmatic disease by treatment with allergenic extracts of clinically significant household inhalants, pollens or molds.

The avoidance or minimization, where possible, of allergens such as house dust in a dust free room, is best illustrated by the goal of attaining the neatest room in the neighborhood.

Bring the allergic equilibrium back into balance:

Allergic Load VS Tolerance

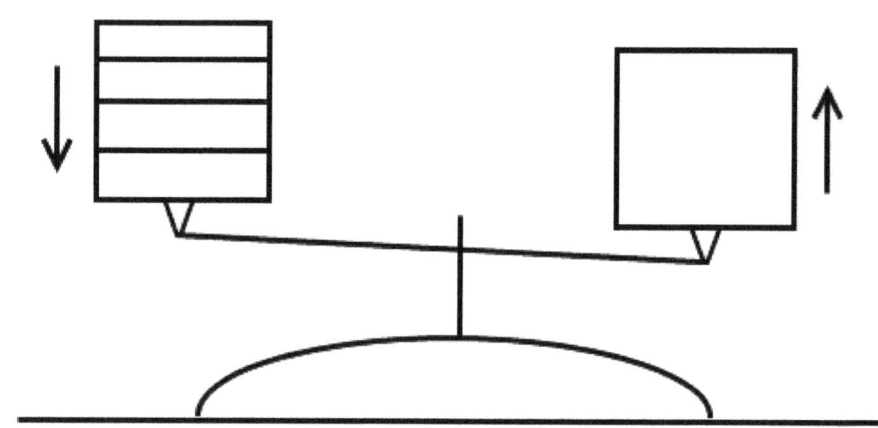

Compromise, minimize and do what is doable in reducing the allergic load.

If the symptomtology is to be reduced or eliminated, it is necessary to make the bedroom as dust-free as possible. The dust-free bedroom should be a room with a minimum number of dust-collecting surfaces and lint-producing fabrics. This does not preclude a cheerful and habitable room. Many things can be done in the room to make it attractive and livable. Decorative wall paper, murals (but no pictures and frames) and bright tile floors (not carpeting) make a cheerful bedroom geared to the allergic patient.

In cleaning the house it is important to use a damp cloth and mop to prevent the spreading of dust allergens.

The filter must be changed monthly in the heater/Air Conditioner. A similar filter should be installed over the vent in the bedroom, which should also be changed monthly. If the window is kept open, a filter screen should be used in the window to keep outdoor pollen, mold and dust from entering the bedroom (a foam screen can be cut to the size of the window and stapled to the screen) or purchased in an appliance hardware store.

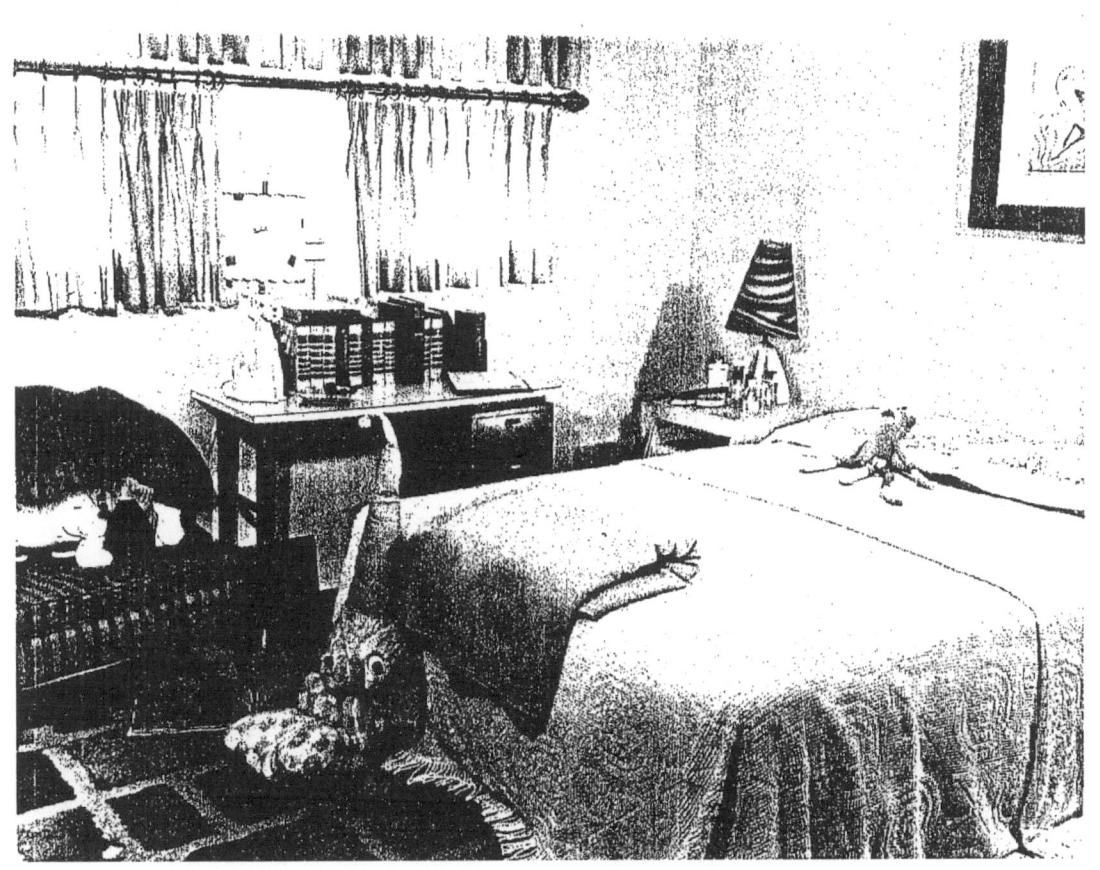

Before

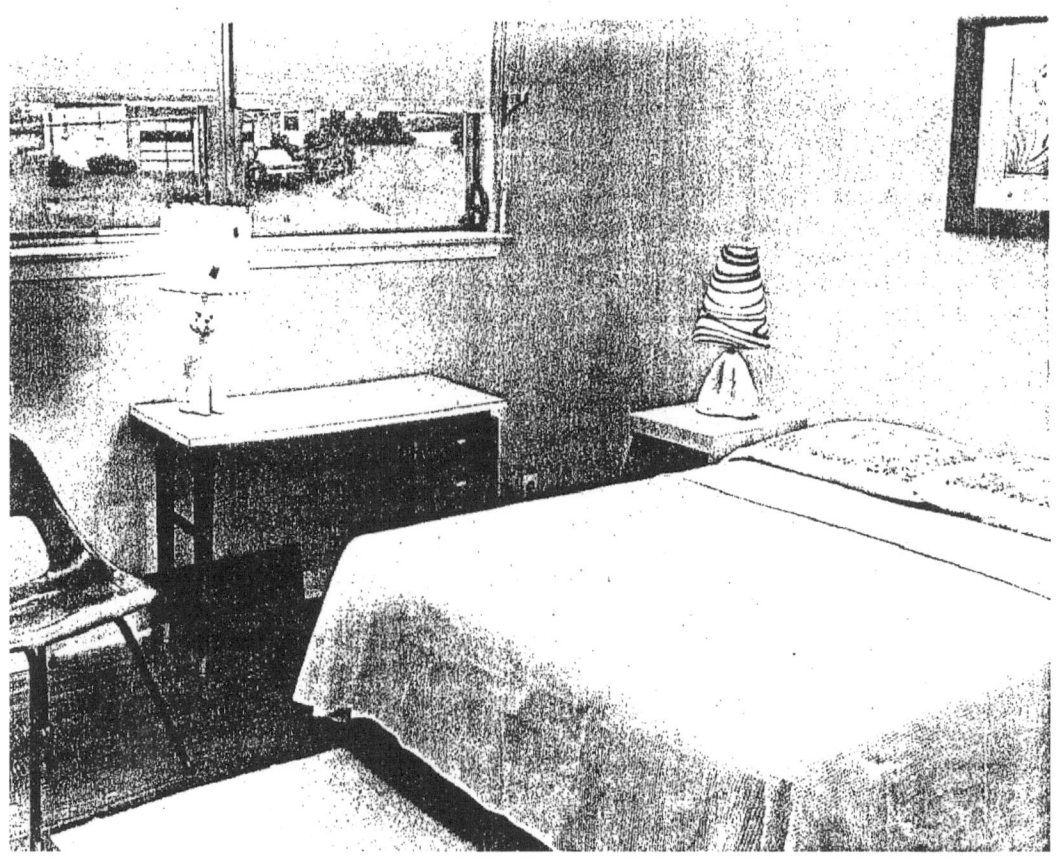

After

We have achieved the goal of attaining the neatest room in the neighborhood.

CONCLUSION

Progressively building from our summary of sports exercise and asthma treatment program, we have:

1. Reinforced the chest muscular pumping action of breathing by breathing exercises associated with sports warm up exercises.

2. Maintained the four minute rule of brief rest after 4 minute spurts of exercise.

3. Practiced and incorporated pursed lip breathing in our practice program.

CONCLUSION, continued

4. Countered and provided further relief through cupped hand percussion and postural drainage providing relief from other obstructive factors by helping the patient to cough up plugs of mucus.

5. Given techniques of breathing, supporting chest muscles and properly coughing up plugs of mucus all of which should be augmented with drinking plenty of fluids and also adhering to dietary and environmental measures along with adequate rest, to prevent aggravating the open airways.

6. **All accomplished with the exciting winning spirit of sports applied to respiratory conditions such as asthma.**

Additional Applications

It seems logical to extend these beneficial effects to adults as well as children and to strengthen the efficiency of muscular function in other medical conditions. This even includes the most challenging of all chronic conditions. The cerebral palsy patients, for example, with varying degrees of limitation can also coordinate their physical therapy with sports warm-up exercises as designed in this book, in the sport of their choice.

"SMOOTH SAILING"

EPILOGUE

Exemplified by some of the patients' art as gifted tokens of appreciation to me as their treating physician-allergist, noting how worthwhile these goals and aspirations are:

The goals and aspirations that help and lead to recovery were expressed by our patients through their art which symbolized their recovery and its processes.

The Smiling Clown. Symbolizing our "encouraging smile," so important an exercise - that aids recovery exemplified in title as one of the paintings.

A Teenager's Celebration of Recovery From Asthma, Expressed in Her Artistic Collage of Her Participation in Many Sports

A collage of many sports painted by one of our patients who could then enjoy and participate in them, after our specialized allergy and immunology care, along with our sports program, was proudly presented to me by this 14 year-old young lady.

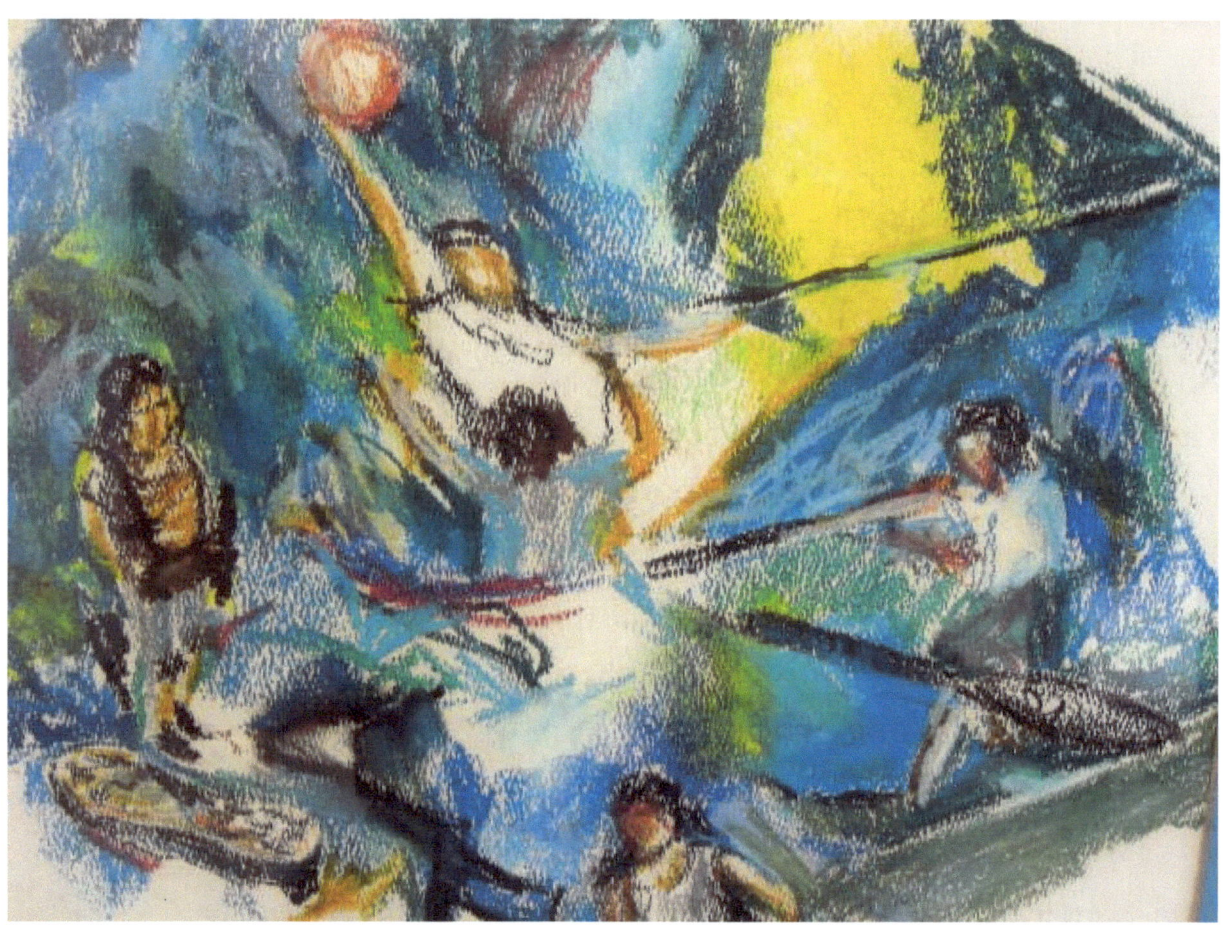

A Patient's Artistic Expression of Immunization and the Thermodynamics of Allergenic Vaccine Production in Allergy Care

A Mandala, (a painting that radiates from the center so that it may be viewed from any angle and always appears upright), expressing all the steps leading to her recovery. This is another allergic patient's artistic interpretation expressing the progressive steps in her care and gratitude for attaining her recovery. The surrounding environmental factors form the four sides of this painting. Her artistic expression shows these environmental allergenic factors, radiating from a central energy, simulating the rays of the sun.

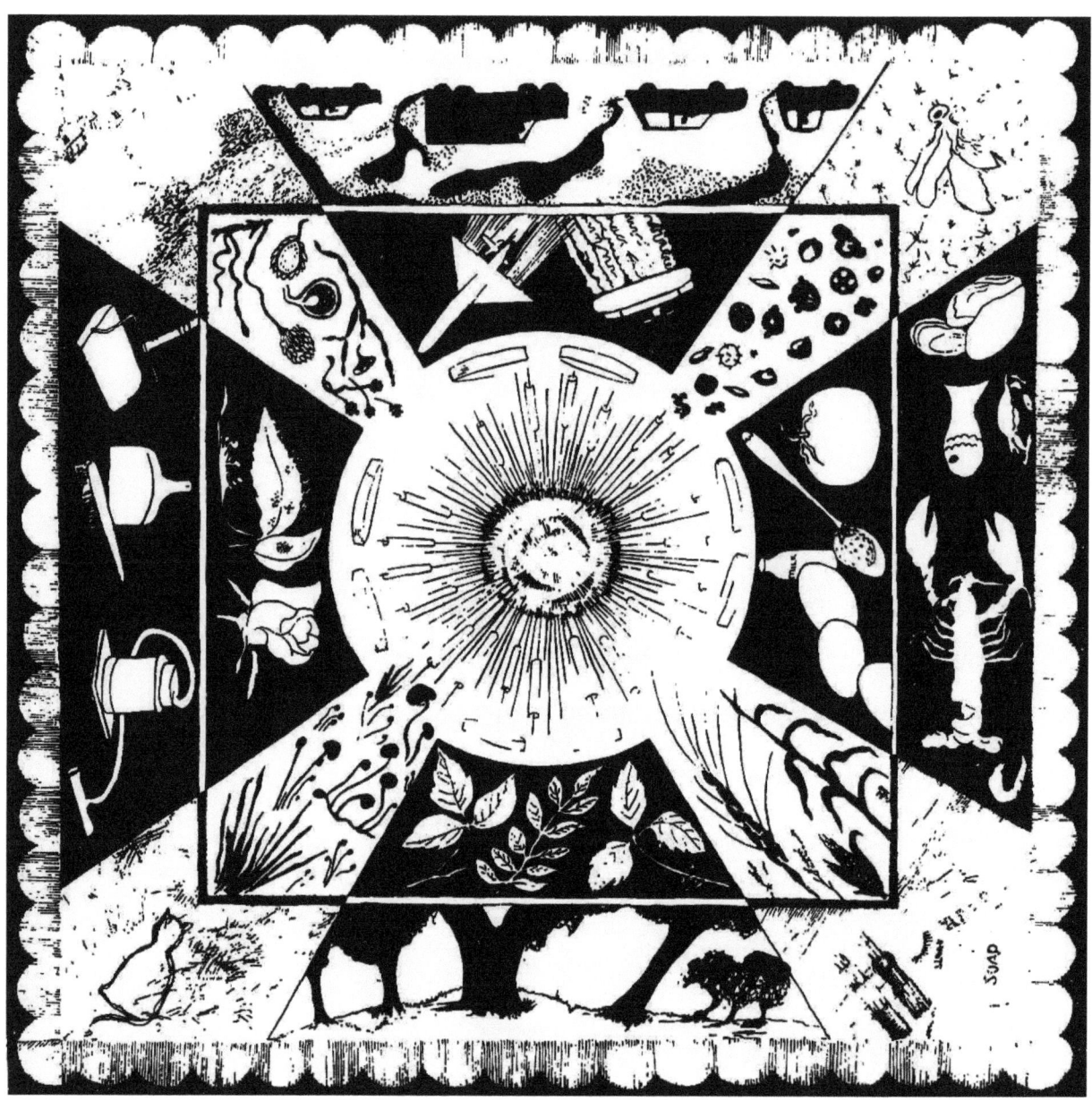

An Allergy Mandela   Margaret L. Hill 1980

A Parent's Celebration of Her Child's Recovery, Through Art

Never before have I seen art that expresses the joy of recovery. Years later, I found through Woody Crumbo's family, he reflects on his work as: "blessing into every piece".

Blue Deer, by Woody Crumbo, described as "Deer Jumping Over the Moon" as a parent's expression of appreciation and delight for her child's recovery. In this painting, we see delight expressed in the skipping and jumping of the deer. When I received the painting as a gift, I told her, "This is also how you made me feel in recounting this recovery."

This parent, working in Woody Crumbo's studio, personally created this silk-screen reproduction.

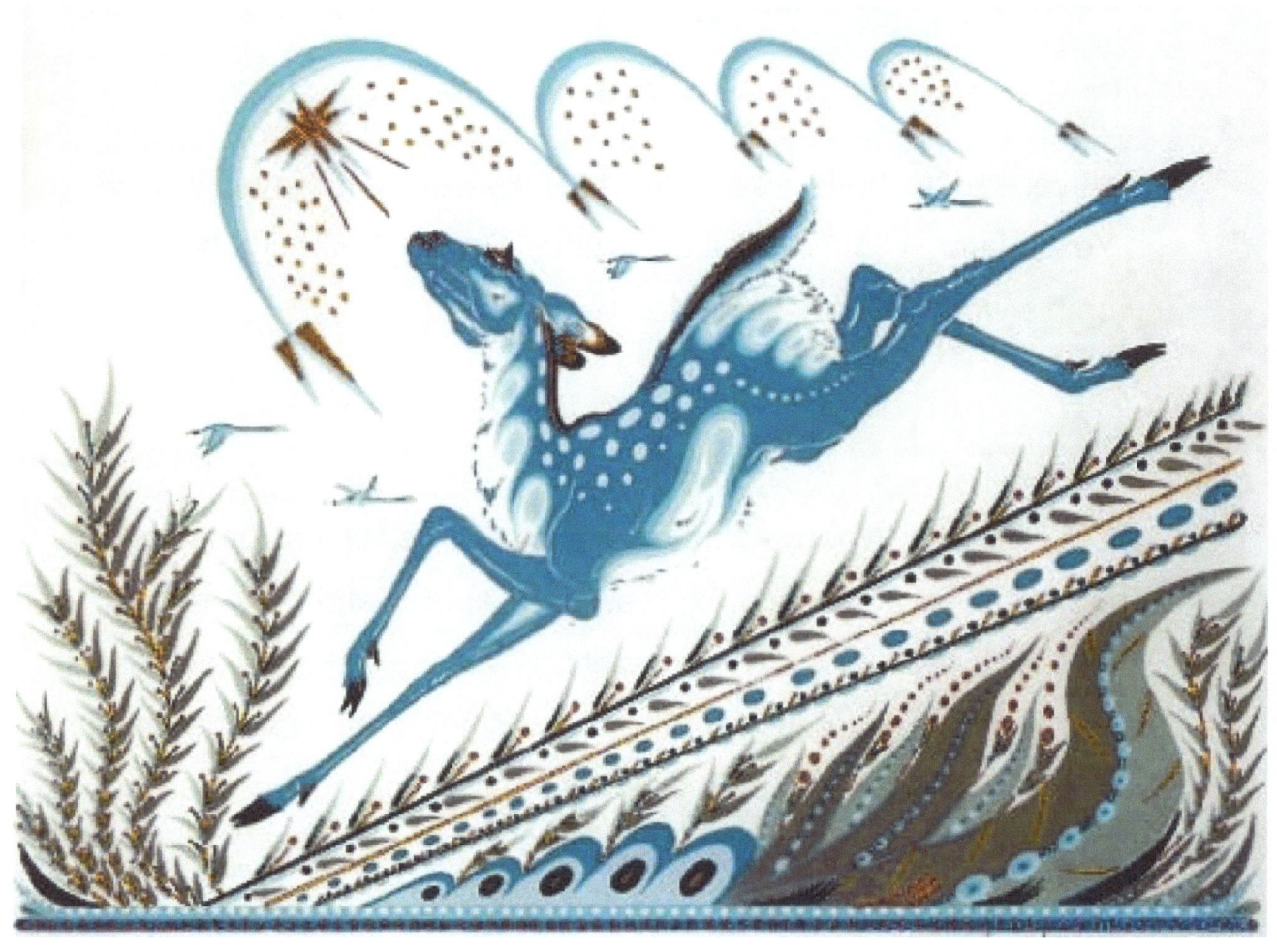

Blue Deer (from the Action Horse Series)
Woody Crumbo 1952

Serigraph on construction paper
reproduced with special permission from Minisa Crumbo-Halsey

LEONARD S. GIRSH, M.D.

Sports, Exercise, & Asthma offers a more complete program in management of Asthma

All part of the Esprit de Corps of the Art of Medicine

(Winning Spirit of the Team)

The healing arts with community support through sports and physical education

Documentation of the world literature in regard to detailed clinical studies in sports, exercise and asthma provides complete confirmation of the clinical evidence. Further confirmative studies: in the experimental animal model of asthma, physical activity also provides documented anti-inflammatory efficacy.

"The thought of being able to engage a child or an adult, in chronic care self management goals, using a favorite sport related warm-up exercise is brilliant in its simplicity and yet can be comprehensive in its outcome." Mark Sobiski, Development Manager Care South Carolina Inc.

"*The Thought Behind the Shot*, admittedly based only upon the Introduction, my impression is WOW. What an encouraging perspective in the treatment of asthmatic patients. Rather than passively and fearfully waiting for an attack, your approach appears to proactively empower your patients and restore joyful activity to children." – A reviewer

In summary, our clinical studies of sports and exercise applied to asthmatic children were met with great success, as well as enthusiastic adherence to the program to meet the goals.

Documentation
For the Medical Profession,
Sports Educators and Asthmatic Patients

Sports, Exercise and Health, **accentuates the development of the accessory muscles of respiration and the detailed development basis of pursed-lip breathing. Training children and adults to breathe with pursed-lips, when necessary, allows for prolonged maintenance of the airway upon expiration to prevent air trapping and collapse of the tracheobronchial tree. Conditioning the patient through this sports exercise training program enables the patient to best cope with and prevent the anxiety mechanism associated with an asthmatic attack.**

The following references support our clinical studies. I initiated this work in several hundred patients, several decades ago while a Professor of Internal Medicine, Allergy and Asthma and as Director of the Pediatric Allergy and Asthma program at Temple University Children's Medical Center and College of Medicine.

Synopsis of advances applying this technology

I.   Physical training is well tolerated, leads to improvements in cardiopulmonary fitness and is not associated with adverse outcomes in people with asthma.

Nineteen studies (695 participants) were included in this review. Physical training was well tolerated (Chandratilleke MG, 2012). There is evidence available to suggest that **physical training has a positive effect on health-related quality of life**, with four studies producing a statistically and **clinically significant benefit with Sports, Exercise and Health.**

104

II.   Randomized controlled trials of breathing retraining in patients of all ages with a diagnosis of asthma. **Retraining of breathing should be a major component of the treatment intervention**.

Improvement, notably in quality of life measurements, are encouraging and well adapted to this program, tabulated data reviewed in publication by Dr. Timothy Craig for children with asthma, all presented here. The bronchopulmonary effects are associated with the comparable benefits of the treadmill in cardiovascular disease.

The mechanism is a reduction of inflammation with clinical improvement in the animal studies, exercise appears to reduce severity and frequency of asthma attacks. **These experiments with mice showed that exercise had an anti-inflammatory effect with significant reduction of production of inflammatory chemicals.**

Lochte and Craig, <u>both focus and concur concerning results of inactivity in asthma</u>, adding an exercise program to the asthmatic patient inactivity and its functional damage to these children and the use of **<u>graduated exercise program to reverse the complications of inactivity.</u>**

The asthmatic children had consistently low predicted aerobic capacity (PAC) when observed across time. Physical activity was positively associated with significant improvement in predicted aerobic capacity in the asthmatics (Lochte, 2012).

To compare longitudinally predicted aerobic capacity of asthmatic children against that of healthy controls during ten months. Methods. Twenty-eight asthmatic children aged 7-15 years and 27 matched controls each performed six sub-maximal exercise tests on treadmill, which included a test of EIA (exercise-induced asthma) (Lochte, 2012).

Children with asthma often experienced breathlessness during physical activity and therefore, unfortunately, tended to avoid vigorous physical activity with disadvantageous consequences to their physical conditioning. There are few pediatric pulmonary conditions in which physical activity has had such potentially harmful effect on patients, limiting exercise capacity (Lochte, 2012).

Predicted aerobic capacity $(mLO(2)/min/kg)$ was calculated. Spirometry and development were measured. Physical activity, medication, and "ever asthma/current asthma" were reported by questionnaire. Predicted aerobic capacity of asthmatics was lower than that of controls $(P = 0.0015)$ across observation times and for both groups an important increase in predicted aerobic capacity according to time was observed $(P < 0.001)$. FEV(1) of the asthmatic children and was within normal range. The majority (86%) of the asthmatics reported pulmonary symptoms to accompany their physical activity. Physical activity (hours per week) showed important effects for the variation in predicted aerobic capacity at baseline $(F = 2.28, P = 0.061)$ and at the T4 observation $(F = 3.03, P = 0.027)$ and the analyses showed important asthma/control group effects at baseline, month four, and month ten. Physical activity of the asthmatics correlated positively with predicted aerobic capacity (Lochte, 2012).

The Vicious Cycle of Inactivity - Individuals with asthma often actively avoid exercise due to symptoms. In one poll, 52% of asthmatic individuals indicated that their health limits their participation in activities, including recreational outdoor sports, going to the gym, and normal physical exertion (e.g. walking up stairs). This same poll found that 40% of adults and 26% of children avoid sports and other exercise induced bronchial spasm activities because of their exercise-induced bronchospasm (EIB) symptoms. This long-term avoidance ultimately results in physical deconditioning. Thus, exercise becomes more difficult with time, and patients become increasingly frustrated with their EIB symptoms, causing them to continue their avoidance (Craig, 2013).

This phenomenon is all the more concerning because of increasing data revealing correlations between obesity and asthma incidence. In addition, there is evidence that inhaled corticosteroids may not be as effective in controlling asthma symptoms in obese patients as they are in normal weight patients. **Given these data and the overall benefits of regular exercise, we believe that it is reasonable to recommend exercise to asthmatic patients., Health care practitioners can help their patients break the cycle of inactivity through education, support, guidance, and optimal control of their underlying asthma** (Craig, 2013).

In conclusion, EIB (Exercise-induced bronchospasm) is a common phenomenon, especially in asthmatic patients and elite athletes. **Data from mouse models demonstrate that exercise down-regulates inflammatory mediators and up-regulates suppressive Treg (T Regulatory Cells) responses. Studies reveal trends of increased QOL (Quality of Life) scores and improved cardiopulmonary fitness in patients after**

undergoing an exercise training program, although this effect is not unique to asthma patients and can be seen in the general population. Numerous other health benefits of an active lifestyle, is reason enough to recommend regular exercise to all patients, including asthmatic patients (Craig, 2013)**.**

We have found that education and motivation along with breathing exercises are the basis for a successful program. An unexpected response emphasizing the success of this program is the fact that even children without asthma were anxious to be included.

The winning spirit of sports with the goal of being able to participate is extended here.

Table 1

Summary of the systemic review by Pacheco, Silva, Alexandrino, Torres.					
Study	**Quality of Life score**	**No. of patients**	**Type**	**Frequency and duration**	**Results**
Children					
Basaran, 2006	Pediatric Asthma Quality of Life Questionnaire	62	Aerobic, moderate	1 hour 3 times per week for 8 weeks	**Significant improvement in both Exercise Group and Controls, but improvement was higher in Exercise Group (P < .001)**
Fanelli, 2007	Pediatric Asthma Quality of Life Questionnaire	38	Aerobic to 70%	1.5 hours 2 times per week for 16 weeks	**Significant improvement in Exercise Group over Control for activity limitation (P < .03), symptoms (P < .02), and emotions (P < 0.03)**
Flapper, 2008	Quality of life Questionnaire	36	Aerobic	2.5 hours once per week for 12 weeks	**Significant improvement in Exercise Group over Control for asthma (P < .023) and DUX-25 (P < .02) scores**
Moreira, 2008	Pediatric Asthma Quality of Life Questionnaire	34	Aerobic	50 minutes 2 times per week for 12 weeks	**Significant improvement in Exercise Group for all domains and non-significant trend in toward improvement in Exercise Group for activity but not different from Control**

Study	Quality of Life score	No. of patients	Type	Frequency and duration	Results
Adults					
Turner, 2010	Asthma Quality of Life Questionnaire	34	Aerobic, moderate	1.5 hours 3 times per week for 6 weeks	**Significant improvement in Exercise Group for total score, activity limitation (P ¼ .04) and symptoms (P ¼ .001)**
Goncalves, 2008	Quality of Life Escola Paulista de Medicina	20	Aerobic to 70%	0.5 hour 2 times per week for 12 weeks	**Significant improvement in Exercise Group over Control for total score (P < .001), activity limitation (P < .001), symptoms (P ¼ .002), and psychosocial (P ¼ .003)**
Mendes, 2010	Quality of Life - Escola Paulista de Medicina	101	Aerobic to 70%	0.5 hour 2 times per week for 12 weeks	**Significant improvement (P < .001) in Exercise Group for total score, activity limitation, symptoms, and psychosocial**

Table 2

Summary of the Cochrane meta-analysis by Chandratilleke MG, Carson KV, Picot J, Brinn MP, Esterman AJ, Smith BJ.			
Study	**Measured outcomes**	**No. of patients**	**Results**
Quality of Life			
Fanelli, 2007	Pediatric Asthma Quality of Life Questionnaire scores	38	**Significant improvement in quality of life**
Turner, 2010	Asthma Quality of Life Questionnaire	35	**Significant improvement in quality of life**
Turner, 2010	Medical Outcomes Study Symptom Free scores	35	**Significant improvement in quality of life**
Mendes, 2010	Quality of Life Escola Paulista de Medicina scores	101	**Significant improvement in quality of life**
Goncalves, 2008	Quality of Life Escola Paulista de Medicina scores	23	**Significant improvement in quality of life**
Moreira, 2008	Pediatric Asthma Quality of Life Questionnaire scores	34	No difference
Cardiopulmonary Fitness			
Ahmaidi, 1993, Cochrane, 1990; Counil, 2003; van Veldhoven, 2001; Varray, 1991; Varray, 1995	maximum oxygen consumption	149	**Mean increase 5.57 mL/kg/min**
Cochrane, 1990; Counil, 2003; van Veldhoven, 1991; Varray, 2001	maximum expiratory volume	111	**Mean increase 6.00 L/min**
Ahmaidi, 1993; Varray, 1991	maximum heart rate	34	**Mean increase 3.67/min**

Study	Measured outcomes	No. of patients	Results
Asthma Symptoms			
Gonçalves, 2008; Mendes, 2010; Mendes, 2011	Symptom-free days	151	**Significant improvement**
Turner, 2010	Asthma Quality of Life Questionnaire scores	35	No difference
Swann, 1983	Daily symptom scores	27	No difference
Varray, 1991	Frequency of attacks	14	No difference
Pulmonary Function			
Moreira, 2008; van Veldhoven, 2001; Varray, 1991; Wang, 2009	forced vital capacity	122	No difference
Mendes, 2011; van Veldhoven, 2001; Wang, 2009; Weisgerber, 2003	peak expiratory flow rate	153	No difference

References

I. Chandratilleke MG, Carson KV, Picot J, Brinn MP, Esterman AJ, Smith BJ. Physical training for asthma. Cochrane Database Syst Rev. 2012 May 16;5:CD001116. doi: 10.1002/14651858.CD001116.pub3.

II. Craig TJ, Dispenza MC. Benefits of exercise in asthma. Ann Allergy Asthma Immunol. 2013 Mar;110(3):133-140.e2. doi: 10.1016/j.anai.2012.10.023.

III. Holloway E, Ram FS. Breathing exercises for asthma. Cochrane Database Syst Rev. 2004;(1):CD001277.

IV. Lochte L. Predicted aerobic capacity of asthmatic children: a research study from clinical origin. Pulm Med. 2012;2012:854652. doi: 10.1155/2012/854652. Epub 2012 Jul 26.

The White House, through Michelle Obama, regarding her national campaign to increase activity and advance diet to counter obesity in children, appreciated that The Thought Behind the Shot be used in this national presentation. Conditioning, using this application technology, can prepare a patient to prevent an asthmatic attack. Breathing exercises and warm-up exercises of their sport of choice enhances the function and activation of the sensory muscles and respiration of the asthmatic child. Based on the observation that musicians playing wind instruments rarely had asthma, this gives the additional positive effects of these exercises.

THE WHITE HOUSE
WASHINGTON

We would like to extend our deepest thanks and appreciation for your generous gift.

It is gratifying to know that we have your support. As we work to address the great challenges of our time, we hope you will continue to stay active and involved.

Again, thank you for your kind gift.

Barack Obama   Michelle Obama

WWW.WHITEHOUSE.GOV

ACKNOWLEDGEMENTS WITH APPRECIATION

I gratefully acknowledge the support I have had from my wife, Annette, who has been my very faithful editor and advisor, offering continual encouragement in this undertaking. I would also like to thank my staff for their support during this effort.

I would also like to thank a number of my contemporaries for their vast knowledge in their review of my book: Arne Olson, Ph.D. Professor, Dept. of Physical Education, Temple University for his contribution in this wonderful program. Dr. Harold L. Paz, M.D. Dean, CEO, Senior V.P. Penn State Hershey College of Medicine. President and Mrs. Barack Obama, White House, utilizing the sport of the child's choice and warm-up exercise as a motivational activity to also fight childhood obesity.

In appreciation to William Katz, Dr. Arne Olsen and Dr. John Jeka for their strong support in the Sports Education Department at Temple University, that helped make this book possible. **Thereby providing advances of clinical success in sports and exercise applied to respiratory disease as: asthma in children and adults as well as a broad basis in helping healthcare**. Motivational stimulus in including exercise in healthcare.

Working with asthmatic patients we can readily see how this bronchopulmonary pump can have a positive effect in severe oxygen deficiency syndromes such as asthma. We are able to see a similar broad-spectrum application. Now the technology is not only being used for the asthmatic patient but for broad-spectrum use as in high-altitude flight in a pressurized cabin monitoring the oxygenation or as a monitor of critically ill patients in the ICU intensive care in developing the Oximeter.

LeRoy Neiman's permission to use his art contribution and our discussions over the years were gifts to me.   I also extend my appreciation to Woody Crumbo and his family for permission to use one of his paintings. This is the only painting I know of that expresses appreciation for recovery of health through art. This painting was a gift to me from a parent in a celebration of the recovery of her child.

A token of appreciation to the many contributors to the world literature and medical sports documentation by the medical scientists that documented the efficacy of *Sports, Exercise and Health* in their medical publications. To my many professors including Dr. Frank C. Whitmore, Dean of The College of Chemistry and Physics at Penn State University and Dr. George C. Bennett, Professor of Anatomy and Dean of Jefferson Medical College whose lecture on *The Anatomy Lesson of Dr. Nicolaes Tulp* by Rembrandt in initiating my lifelong appreciation of structure and function which inspired me in this direction of advancing medicine.

Appreciation goes to the many patients from different clinics that wanted to join our program making it a success in multiple pediatric disease application.
Finally, the 'university' of my family for the realization that 'a problem is an opportunity in work clothes'.

LEONARD S. GIRSH, M.D.

All about the Author

Dr. Girsh is a Gold Medalist in Clinical Surgery Regenerative medicine and Tissue Engineering graduate of Jefferson Medical College and University, Penn State University School of Chemistry and Physics. He is Boarded in Internal Medicine, Allergy and Pediatrics (Clinical Immunology and Allergy).

Building on these advances, as an Immunochemist, Dr. Girsh developed immunotherapeutics that restores tissue integrity, innate immunity. This was based upon and derived from one of the leading clinical practices on the east coast of Immunology and Allergy applied to Internal Medicine, Pediatrics, and Clinical Surgery, with empathy, dedication and devotion to patient care and recovery.

Sports, Exercise and Health provides a fulfilled wish for the asthmatic, initially dedicated to children, by incorporating the motivational sports exercise of the sport of their choice in the asthmatic patient's program of recovery. Children from other clinics were waiting to enroll even though they did not have asthma. We, of course, accepted them.

His unique therapeutics is derived from clinical and therapeutic experience while in positions of leadership incorporating opportunities of professorships and immunology department directorships at Temple University in Philadelphia, PA, where he founded the Department of Occupational Health based on studies that advanced the treatment of bronchial asthma. He also founded the Asthmatic Center at Children's Heart Hospital, Philadelphia, PA.

He has published more than 50 medical articles and held professorships and immunology department directorships at Temple University in Philadelphia, PA, a visiting professorship at Oxford University, where his clinical studies provided advances in hypoallergenic milk. Dr. Girsh also served as adjunct professor in Life Sciences, University of Wisconsin where he collaborated on a patent in advancing the treatment of intestinal obstruction.

Dr. Girsh was instrumental in establishing one of the first national post-graduate courses in allergy and asthma that focused upon allergic and asthmatic children, presented at Temple University. Additional professorships include a visiting professorship at Oxford University, along with an adjunct professorship in Life Sciences, University of Wisconsin.

His scientific contributions include development in the '50s of what is still the current treatment of lead poisoning, while at Jefferson in collaboration with Riker Pharmaceutical Company.

Dr. Girsh worked to establish an air quality program with scientists at the Franklin Institute, Philadelphia, PA and the Air Quality Division of the City of Philadelphia, which monitors the levels of air quality and pollution. Several years of data collection were utilized tracking the impact of air quality and weather change on the number of hospital admissions of asthmatic children, resulting in the publication of *A Study of the Epidemiology of Asthma in Children in Philadelphia*, and his chairmanship of the Air Pollution and Air Quality Committee, American Academy of Allergy.

Meeting with the industrial leaders of Philadelphia, who at his suggestion, and improved air quality to met EPA standards, most helpful to asthmatic patients.

In collaboration with Hewlett-Packard, he developed the fiber-optic pulse Oximeter. Together he presented this in a series of national scientific exhibits including the Franklin Institute of Philadelphia. These advances have been substantial and sustainable as they are currently in continued use, not only benefiting the medical care of asthmatic patients but also used worldwide in every field of medicine, like the stethoscope. It has also been incorporated as a panel in major hospitals, for which he received nomination for the Lasker-DeBakey Award, currently earns the healthcare industry $3.5 billion annually.

Dr. Girsh was recognized three times by the Four Chaplains Legion of Honor in Philadelphia, PA, for outstanding service to the community. These recommendations came from patients.

Dr. Girsh has served as a consultant for many corporations devoted to advances in medical science and patient care, including special assignments from the Leatherhead Food Research Association (UK) and Wisconsin Alumni Research Foundation.

Dr. Girsh resides with his wife Annette in Naples, Florida, where he practices as a medical consultant along with developing new products in collaboration with the Florida Business and Economic Development Counsel for the advancement of medicine.

PUBLISHER'S NOTE TO READERS

The information in this book can be a valuable addition to your doctor's advice, but it is not intended to replace the services of trained health professionals. You are advised to consult with your doctor regarding matters relating to your health, particularly regarding symptoms that may require immediate attention.

IMPORTANT NOTE TO READERS

The material in this book is for educational purposes and can be a valuable addition to your physician's advice. Please discuss all aspects of *The Thought Behind The Shot* with your physician before beginning this program of exercises with their positive results as shared and reported in this book.